Drug treatment in psychiatry

Trevor Silverstone is Professor of Clinical Psychopharmacology in the University of London at St Bartholomew's Hospital, one of the constituent teaching hospitals of the university. He obtained a degree in physiology at Oxford, trained in medicine at St Bartholomew's Hospital, and in psychiatry at the Maudsley Hospital and the Institute of Psychiatry, London. He has had research experience in neurophysiology, at the University of California, Los Angeles, and in psychopharmacology, at the University of Pennsylvania. Professor Silverstone has published extensively on clinical psychopharmacology in scientific and medical journals. He is the general editor of the Routledge series 'Social and Psychological Aspects of Medical Practice', of which *Drug Treatment in Psychiatry* is the first volume, and editor of *International Clinical Psychopharmacology*.

Paul Turner is Professor of Clinical Pharmacology in the University of London at St Bartholomew's Hospital, and is Honorary Consultant Physician to St Bartholomew's Hospital. After medical training at the Middlesex Hospital, London, and four years' experience in general medicine, Paul Turner set up a department of clinical pharmacology at St Bartholomew's Hospital. His publications include *Clinical Aspects of Autonomic Pharmacology* (Heinemann Medical, 1969) and *Clinical Pharmacology* (Churchill Livingstone, 1985).

**Social and Psychological Aspects
of Medical Practice**

Editor: Trevor Silverstone

Also in this series:

Malcolm Lader
The Psychophysiology of Mental Illness

J. Stuart Whitely and John Gordon
Group Approaches in Psychiatry

S. Gilbert
Pathology of Eating

Drug treatment in psychiatry

FOURTH EDITION

Trevor Silverstone, MA, DM, FRCP, FRCPsych,
Professor of Clinical Psychopharmacology,
St Bartholomew's Hospital, London

Paul Turner, MD, BSC, FRCP
Professor of Clinical Pharmacology,
St Bartholomew's Hospital, London

London and New York

First published in 1974
Second edition 1978
Third edition 1982
Fourth edition 1988
by Routledge
11 New Fetter Lane, London EC4P 4EE

Published in the USA by
Routledge
in association with Routledge, Chapman and Hall, Inc.
29 West 35th Street, New York, NY 10001

Reprinted 1991

Set in 10/12pt Baskerville by
Columns of Reading
and printed in Great Britain by
Richard Clay Ltd, Bungay, Suffolk

British Library Cataloguing in Publication Data
Silverstone, Trevor
   Drug treatment in psychiatry—4th ed.
   —(Social and psychological aspects of medical practice).
   1. Psychopharmacology 2. Mental illness
   —Chemotherapy
   I. Title II. Turner, Paul, 1933–
   III. Series
   616.89'18   RC483

Library of Congress Cataloging in Publication Data
Silverstone, Trevor
   Drug treatment in psychiatry.
   (Social and psychological aspects of medical practice)
   Includes bibliographies and index.
   1. Psychopharmacology. 2. Mental illness—
   Chemotherapy. I. Turner, Paul. II. Title:
   III. Series. [DNLM: 1. Mental Disorders—drug therapy.
   2. Psychopharmacology. WM 402 S587d]
   RC483.S515 1988   616.89'   87-28690

ISBN 0-415-00264-8

Contents

Figures and Tables

Preface to the fourth edition

Since writing the first edition of this book over fourteen years have elapsed. During that time a host of new drugs have been introduced for the treatment of mental illnesses, and some have both come and gone. What has not changed is our principle aim in writing this book: to provide an introduction to psychopharmacology for all those concerned in the management of psychiatric disorders.

Another principle which we have maintained is our conviction that drug therapy should have a sound physiological and pharmacological basis wherever possible. To this end each major clinical chapter begins with a review of current knowledge about the underlying physiological and biochemical factors concerned in the conditions under consideration; this is followed by a description of the pharmacology of the drugs used in clinical treatment. The practical guidelines for treatment which come next can thus be seen in their appropriate scientific context.

Recent developments in clinical psychopharmacology covered in this edition include a full discussion of benzodiazepine dependence and the problems of withdrawal, the place of anticonvulsants in the treatment and prophylaxis of manic–depressive illness and the neuroleptic malignant syndrome. We have also incorporated the classification of diseases put forward by the American Psychiatric Association (*DSM III*) in the clinical sections of the book.

Aging, and the many psychiatric problems associated with it, has become an increasingly important topic, and we have added a new chapter devoted exclusively to it. Partly in order to prevent the book outgrowing its comfortable size and partly to keep the subjects covered within the professional context of most practising psychiatrists we have deleted the chapter on pain. The greater part of the chapter on sexual function has also disappeared, but we have retained the section on sexual deviance, including it in a reorganised chapter entitled 'Substance abuse, personality disorders and sexual deviance'.

Help from our colleagues in the completion of our task has been given unstintingly. We are truly grateful to them all. In addition we wish to express our particular thanks to Irene Fox who typed the manuscript and Emma Turner for preparing the index.

Trevor Silverstone
Paul Turner

General principles

Part I

Historical introduction

1

A desire to take medicine is, perhaps, the great feature which distinguishes man from other animals.

William Osler, 1894

A drug, according to the World Health Organisation, is 'any substance which when taken into the living organism may modify one of its functions'. Psychotropic drugs are those which have, through their action on the brain, an effect on normal and abnormal psychological processes.

Perhaps the first such substance to be discovered, certainly the first to be referred to in Western literature, is alcohol: 'and Noah began to be a husbandman, and he planted a vineyard and he drank of the wine, and was drunken. . . .' In fact it is unlikely that there ever was a time when alcoholic beverages were not used; certainly the Egyptians drank freely of them and there is a picture dating from 1500 BC illustrating the unfortunate effects of drinking to excess. The word itself stems from the Arabic *al kihl* meaning essence, and *alcohol vini* referred to the essential or most subtle part of the wine.

Several other substances which are both used and abused in present-day society have almost as extended a lineage as has alcohol. Opium poppy seeds have been discovered in Stone Age settlements in Switzerland dating from at least 2000 BC. Homer described the action of nepenthe, which most authorities believe to be synonymous with opium, as giving 'forgetfulness of evil'. There is even some suggestion that the secret of opium, probably coming from Egypt, was closely guarded by the elite and was given to certain chosen warriors (heroes) before such epic battles as Troy. The habit of taking opium spread throughout Europe and the East in spite of warnings against intemperate use; until de Quincey, in the early nineteenth century, vividly portrayed the agonies which

3

could come from dependence on it, most Englishmen regarded opium as but a simple family remedy.

Another drug which acts on the central nervous system, known to the ancients and still with us, is marihuana, the derivative of *Cannabis indica*. A Chinese emperor writing in 2200 BC referred to its euphoric properties and advised that its use should be restricted, as in his opinion it was little more than a 'liberator of sin'. Perhaps the most famous users of marihuana, or hashish, were the assassins (whose very name derived from the word hashish), a fanatical thirteenth-century Persian sect who, when intoxicated, would recklessly commit the most brutal murders.

On the other side of the world, in South America, the leaf of the coca tree containing cocaine was, until quite recently, as widely taken by the indigenous peoples of the Andes as alcohol in our society. Unlike alcohol, which is a sedative, cocaine is a central stimulant and allowed the Incas and their descendants to work prodigiously without fatigue. Because of this property its use was encouraged by the Spanish mine-owners.

Even stranger are the effects of *peyotl*, the sacred cactus of Mexico. This contains mescaline, a potent hallucinogenic compound, which so distorts the processes of perception that brilliant dream-like visions may be experienced. More recently other hallucinogenic substances such as lysergic acid diethylamide (LSD) have enjoyed a certain vogue.

The drugs thus far considered have all been taken in the first instance to obtain a state of pleasurable relaxation or contentment; it was only much later that the isolation of the active principle of opium and morphine, in 1817, and of cocaine in 1885, allowed a medicinal application.

An ancient remedy from India, *Rauwolfia serpentina*, which has always been used therapeutically rather than socially, turned out to be of considerable theoretical and practical interest. Indian texts have for three thousand years recommended the root of this plant, which contains reserpine, in cases of psychiatric disturbance, a recommendation which was found in the 1950s to be soundly based, and reserpine was among the first of the newer 'antipsychotic' drugs. Unfortunately its side effects proved unacceptable, and it was superseded as a treatment for psychotic illness by newer, synthetic compounds.

Indeed it was in 1952, the very same year in which reserpine was formally introduced into modern psychiatry, that Delay and

Deniker described the dramatic effect of the wholly synthetic compound chlorpromazine in cases of schizophrenia, and in so doing may be said to have inaugurated the subspeciality of psychopharmacology which has grown so rapidly in recent years. As with many other important therapeutic advances, the use of chlorpromazine was based on a chance observation. Promethazine, an antihistamine drug, was noted to exhibit sedative effects, and chlorpromazine, which is chemically related to promethazine (they are both phenothiazines), was synthesised in the hope of increasing this sedative action. However, it was found that its range of activity was much wider, and it was soon being prescribed for a variety of conditions, particularly schizophrenia and mania.

Shortly after the synthesis and clinical investigation of chlorpromazine another breakthrough came with the discovery of the monoamine oxidase inhibitors. As in the case of chlorpromazine, this also arose out of an unexpected clinical observation, namely that tuberculous patients being treated with iproniazid became rather more euphoric than might have been expected. As a result it was suggested that if iproniazid did have a real mood-elevating action, it might be related to its ability to inhibit the enzyme monoamine oxidase, and thereby affect brain amine concentrations (see chapter 2). If this were so it was further reasoned that such compounds might be of considerable therapeutic benefit in cases of depression. Although iproniazid itself was soon found to be too toxic for widespread application, a variety of other less toxic monoamine oxidase inhibitors have been synthesised, and the introduction of this class of drugs has greatly stimulated investigation into the biochemical basis of depression itself (see chapter 7).

As frequently happens, the discovery of one major new drug like chlorpromazine leads to a hurried search for other members of the same chemical class which, it is hoped will prove more effective than the original compound. In the course of such a search, drugs bearing a superficial structural resemblance to the parent compound may be found to cause clinical effects quite different from those expected. Such was the case with imipramine, which was originally synthesised in the hope of producing an iminodibenzyl derivative related to chlorpromazine with an even stronger sedative action. On clinical trial imipramine had little sedative activity but did exhibit a marked antidepressant activity – a property which had not been forecast. Since then many other drugs in the same group (the tricyclic antidepressants) have been introduced (see chapter 7).

Among the more significant advances to have taken place in recent years has been the confirmation of Cade's earlier report that the element lithium is effective in improving the symptoms of mania. Not only does lithium relieve the acute symptoms, it appears to have a true prophylactic activity in preventing recurrences of both the manic and depressive episodes which occur in those patients who are predisposed to manic–depressive psychosis (see chapter 7).

The newer synthetic drugs thus far considered, the phenothiazines, the monoamine oxidase inhibitors and the tricyclic antidepressants, have all been directed mainly at the more severe forms of psychiatric illness, the psychoses. There remains, however, a great deal of minor psychological distress, mainly manifested as anxiety or the somatic accompaniments of anxiety, which accounts for a considerable proportion of the conditions presenting in general practice and internal medicine. Therefore any drug that can relieve such anxiety symptoms will obviously have a ready appeal. The barbiturates, the first of which, malonylurea (barbituric acid, possibly named in honour of St Barbara), was synthesised in 1864. Although the barbiturates were shown to have significant antianxiety effects, they were also found to be dangerous when taken in overdose, to cause marked enzyme induction in the liver and to cause problems of dependence.

Largely as a result of these undesirable effects the barbiturates came to be almost entirely replaced by benzodiazepine derivatives which were not only much safer but were thought to be free of any dependence-producing potential. Unfortunately this has not turned out to be the case, and benzodiazepine dependence is proving increasingly troublesome (see chapter 8). In order to circumvent this problem, newer non-benzodiazepine antianxiety drugs are being developed.

Since the 1950s when most of the drugs discussed were originally introduced, largely, as we have seen, due to chance, there has been a spate of new variants. There are currently available in the United Kingdom twenty-five antipsychotic compounds, eighteen antidepressants, four monoamine oxidase inhibitors and twelve benzodiazepine compounds. Not only the variety but also the total number of prescriptions for these drugs are rising rapidly.

In a welcome attempt to provide some shape and order in this welter of information, and to assist the study of psychopharmacology generally, a committee of the World Health

Organisation suggested the following classification of psychotropic drugs.

1 *Antipsychotics*: drugs with therapeutic effects on psychoses and other types of psychiatric disorder. In addition they frequently produce extrapyramidal effects, such as tremor and rigidity.

2 *Antidepressants*: drugs effective in the treatment of pathological depressive states.

3 *Antianxiety drugs*: substances that reduce pathological anxiety, tension and agitation, without therapeutic effect on disturbed cognitive or perceptual processes. These drugs usually raise the convulsive threshold and do not produce extrapyramidal or autonomic effects. They may produce drug dependence.

4 *Psychostimulants*: drugs that increase the level of alertness and/or motivation.

5 *Psychodysleptics*: drugs producing abnormal mental phenomena, particularly in the cognitive and perceptual spheres.

More recently a further class of psychotropic drugs has been developed.

6 *Nooceptive drugs*: drugs which improve cognitive function and memory.

The above classification will be used throughout this book. The first part of the book deals with the general principles underlying the pharmacological activity of psychotropic drugs within the central nervous system; the various pharmacokinetic considerations which can influence the intensity and duration of such activity; the ways in which the effects of psychotropic drugs can be monitored in man; the social and psychological factors which affect the acceptance of, and response to, psychotropic drugs.

The second part of the book is organised clinically, and contains a series of chapters relating to the various clinical conditions seen in psychiatric practice. The classification of clinical syndromes used in this book is based largely on the scheme set out in the third edition of *The Diagnostic and Statistical Manual of the American*

Psychiatric Association (DSM III). The compounds are discussed in association with the various conditions covered. Each of those chapters consists of an introduction to the underlying physiology and pathology of the given conditions (as far as they are known); this is followed by a discussion of the pharmacology of the various drugs used in their treatment; in the final section a recommended therapeutic approach, using the drugs already discussed, is presented.

Suggestions for further reading

AMERICAN PSYCHIATRIC ASSOCIATION, *Diagnostic and Statistical Manual III*, American Psychiatric Association, Washington DC, 1986.

AYD, F., and BLACKWELL, B., *Discoveries in Biological Psychiatry*, Lippincott, Philadelphia, 1970.

INGLIS, B., *The Forbidden Game, A Social History of Drugs*, Hodder & Stoughton, London, 1975.

IVERSEN, S., *Psychopharmacology: Recent Advances and Future Prospects*, Oxford University Press, Oxford, 1985.

JOHNSON, F. N., and CADE, J. F. J., 'The historical background to lithium research and therapy', in *Lithium Research and Therapy*, ed. F. N. Johnson, Academic Press, London, 1975.

LEWIN, L., *Phantastica – Narcotic and Stimulating Drugs, Their Use and Abuse*, Routledge & Kegan Paul, London, 1931 (reprinted 1964).

LIPTON, M. A., DI MASCIO, A., and KILLAM, K. F., *Psychopharmacology: A Generation of Progress*, Raven Press, New York, 1978.

SWAZEY, J. P., *Chlorpromazine in Psychiatry, A Study of Therapeutic Innovation*, MIT Press, Cambridge, Mass., 1974.

WORLD HEALTH ORGANISATION, *Research in Psychopharmacology*, WHO Technical Report, series no. 371, 1967.

Pharmacology of central nervous system transmission   2

Neurohumoral transmission

The effects of drugs on mood, perception and consciousness can best be understood in terms of their actions on the underlying chemical mechanisms responsible for normal function of the central nervous system.

The contacts between one nerve cell and another within the central nervous system as well as in the peripheral autonomic ganglia are called 'synapses'. This term was first introduced by Sherrington in 1897 and is derived from the Greek word *synopsis*, meaning 'clasp'. It reflects the intimate nature of the contact between cells, which Sherrington, like others before him, recognised to be present.

The mechanism by which nerve impulses are propagated from one cell across the synapse to the other was a matter of considerable controversy until the middle of this century. According to one school of thought, synaptic transmission could be explained solely in terms of electrical events, whereas a second school of thought maintained that nerve impulses were transmitted by chemical substances released from the nerve endings. This idea was strengthened at the turn of the century by the observations of Lewandowsky and Langley that injection of extracts from adrenal glands produced similar effects in experimental animals to stimulation of sympathetic nerves. Elliott, in 1904, suggested that sympathetic nerve impulses released minute amounts of an adrenaline-like substance in close contact with the effector cells. In 1907, Dixon drew attention to the close similarity between the effects of the alkaloid muscarine and responses to vagal stimulation, and put forward the hypothesis that such stimulation liberated a muscarine-like substance, which acted as a chemical transmitter of the impulses to the effector cell. It was not until

1921, however, that Loewi demonstrated that stimulation of the vagus nerve of one frog heart released a substance into the perfusion fluid which slowed the rate of a second heart when the perfusion fluid flowed through it. Loewi and Navratil went on to show that this substance was acetylcholine.

It is now generally agreed that transmission at most, if not all, synapses in the mammalian central nervous system is mediated by chemical agents. These are released by action potentials which pass down the axon, and interact with receptors on the post-synaptic effector cell body to increase its permeability to ions and set up a further action potential within it.

Before a compound can be considered to be a neurochemical transmitter it should conform to the following criteria:

1 it must be present in the nerve endings
2 the neurone must contain the enzymes necessary for its manufacture and release
3 the presence of various precursors in the synthetic pathway should be demonstrable
4 there should be systems for the inactivation of the transmitter; where enzymes are involved, they should be demonstrable within the neurone or in its immediate vicinity
5 during nerve stimulation the substance should be detectable in extracellular fluid collected from the region of the activated synapses
6 when applied to the post-synaptic cell body the substance should mimic the action of the synaptically released transmitter
7 drugs which are thought to produce their effect by interaction within the transmitter should be shown to interact with it in the predicted manner under experimental conditions

The last two criteria are probably the most important.

The bodies of nerve cells in the central nervous system are densely covered by synapses, and it is probable that they have more than one transmitter substance acting on their surfaces. It has been shown, for example, that at least three transmitters act on one type of cell, the Renshaw cell in the spinal cord, two of them being excitatory transmitters and one an inhibitory transmitter. Other experiments have shown that neurones in the cerebral cortex are inhibited by at least two distinct transmitter substances.

When it is recalled how difficult it was to demonstrate neurohumoral transmission in relatively simple peripheral synapses, and that it is only in recent years that all the seven criteria listed above have been satisfied for them, the difficulties of unequivocally demonstrating transmitter substances in the central nervous system will be appreciated. In fact, the evidence for most of the substances which have been postulated to act in the central nervous system is only circumstantial and fulfils but a few of these criteria.

Among the substances suggested are:

Acetylcholine   Gamma-aminobutyric acid
Noradrenaline   Glycine and taurine
Adrenaline   Glutamic and aspartic acids
5-hydroxytryptamine   Peptides
Histamine   Prostaglandins
                                 Cyclic nucleotides

Acetylcholine

Acetylcholine together with appropriate enzymes for its synthesis and degradation is widely present in the central nervous system. Histochemical studies have revealed probable cholinergic pathways to the cerebral cortex in the ascending reticular system partly from the N. basalis of Meynert and in the cerebellum. Microinjection techniques using iontophoresis have shown that neurones sensitive to acetylcholine are present in all regions of the central nervous system. In the spinal cord acetylcholine produces only excitation of neuronal activity, but in other parts of the central nervous system and brain both excitatory and inhibitory effects may be seen. The effects of acetylcholine in the spinal cord seem to be mainly nicotinic, while those in the cerebral cortex are predominantly muscarinic, and can be blocked by antimuscarinic agents such as atropine and hyoscine. The central effects of these drugs differ, atropine having excitant and hyoscine depressant actions, and they probably depend on their anticholinergic effects on different groups of neurones in the brain.

ATROPINE ⟶ (M) ⟶ EXCITATION
HYOSCINE ⟶ (M) ⟶ DEPRESSANT.

Noradrenaline (norepinephrine)

Noradrenaline (NA) unlike acetylcholine, is not widely distributed throughout the central nervous system but is concentrated in the hypothalamus and brain stem (Figure 1). There are two major groups of NA containing cell bodies from which axonal systems

11

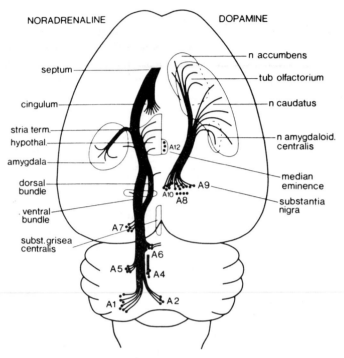

NORADRENALINE   DOPAMINE

Horizontal projection of the ascending NA and DA pathways

Figure 1 *The distribution of noradrenergic and dopaminergic pathways in the brain* (after U. Ungerstedt, *Acta Physiologica Scandinavica Supplement* no. 367, 1971)

arise to innervate other areas throughout the brain via the dorsal and ventral noradrenergic bundles. The largest of these two groups is the locus coeruleus, so called because of the pigment which the cells contain in man and the higher primates. Electrophysiological activation of this pathway produces inhibition of spontaneous discharge in the areas which it innervates, particularly the cerebellum, hippocampus and cerebral cortex, the receptors involved having the pharmacological characteristics of beta-adrenoceptors (page 25). The second group of neurones are less well defined and are scattered throughout the lateral tegmental system. Their physiological and pharmacological activities have not yet been defined.

Adrenaline (epinephrine)

There is evidence that a neuronal system exists in the medullary and hypothalmic nuclei concerned with autonomic control in which adrenaline is the neurotransmitter. Its functional role is still uncertain.

Dopamine

Dopamine is a precursor in the synthetic pathway of NA:

Phenylalanine – tyrosine – dopa – dopamine – noradrenaline

It is not surprising, therefore, that it should be present in the brain in about the same amount as NA. It does not have the same distribution, however. Fluorescent studies have shown that dopamine is particularly localised in (a) the nigro-striatal area, with projections into the limbic cortex and other limbic structures (the mesolimbic system); (b) the tuberoinfundibular system which links periventricular nuclei with the intermediate lobe of the pituitary and median eminence; (c) the medulla, with dopaminergic cells associated with nuclei of the vagus nerve and the nucleus tractus solitarius.

It is convenient, on anatomical and functional grounds, to subdivide the dopaminergic system into five functional pathways:

1 *Nigro-striatal pathway* A deficiency of dopamine in this system produces a clinical syndrome characterised by involuntary movements and disordered muscle tone and coordination. This occurs in Parkinson's disease, and may be produced by drugs which deplete the brain of dopamine, such as reserpine, or block dopamine receptors, such as phenothiazines or butyrophenones. The effects of dopamine in the basal ganglia are opposed by acetylcholine and other muscarinic agents. One such compound, tremorine, produces a parkinsonian-like tremor in experimental animals which can be abolished by atropine and related drugs. The effectiveness of anticholinergic drugs such as benzhexol (Artane) and orphenadrine (Disipal) in the treatment of Parkinson's disease is probably due to their ability to block these central effects of acetylcholine.

2 *Hypothalamic–hypophyseal pathway* Dopamine is released from the neurones of this pathway, and inhibits prolactin release.

13

Prolactin secretion results in an increase in activity of these neurones by an action within the hypothalamus. Drugs which deplete the brain of dopamine or block dopamine receptors release the anterior pituitary from its inhibitory action and result in hyperprolactinaemia. Dopamine receptor agonists, such as bromocriptine, which stimulate these pituitary receptors, inhibit prolactin secretion in a similar way to dopamine.

3 *Mesolimbic pathway* It is possible that the affective disorders and schizophrenia are associated with disorders of this system.

4 *Mesocortical pathway* This pathway is possibly involved in the pathogenesis of drug-induced akathisia.

5 *Medullary pathway* Dopamine is closely involved in emetic activity, dopamine agonists such as bromocriptine commonly producing vomiting, and antagonists such as phenothiazines and metoclopramide being effective antiemetics. It is possible that the medullary dopaminergic pathway is associated with emesis.

5-Hydroxytryptamine (serotonin)

Like NA, 5-hydroxytryptamine (5–HT) is concentrated mainly in the hypothalamus and brain stem. Neurones in the mid-brain raphé nuclei containing 5–HT show a yellow fluorescence in contrast to the green of NA containing neurones. 5–HT secreting neurones are thought to extend from the brain stem into the cerebral cortex and hippocampal areas.

Electrophysiological studies indicate that activation of these 5–HT pathways produces mainly inhibitory effects in the target areas which they innervate. 5–HT has widespread effects on vegetative functions such as appetite, sleep and sexual behaviour.

Hallucinogenic drugs and 5–HT Studies carried out around 1950 suggested that the potent hallucinogen LSD might produce its behavioural effects by antagonising the action of 5–HT in the brain, as it does in some smooth muscle preparations such as the rat uterus. Neuropharmacological studies carried out since that time have shown that this is too simplistic a view, however, and that while 5–HT neurones may be involved in the action of some

14

hallucinogenic drugs, no consistent pattern of 5–HT antagonism or potentiation has yet been demonstrated.

Histamine

Histamine can be found in synaptic vesicles in the hypothalamus, thalamus and cortex. Intraventricular injections of histamine produce changes in the cortical EEG and a state of sedation in experimental animals. Microinjection studies have shown that it depresses the excitatory threshold of neurones in the spinal cord, and has both depressant and excitant effects on neurones in the cerebral cortex. Its precursor histidine, from which it is formed by a simple one-step decarboxylation, has a depressant action on cortical neurones.

The actions of histamine throughout the body appear to be mediated by two types of receptor, designated H_1 and H_2. The H_1 effects are contraction of smooth muscle of the intestine, bronchioles, uterus and large blood vessels, dilation of small blood vessels, especially venules, and increasing vascular permeability to plasma proteins. The most important H_2 receptor effect is stimulation of the acid-secreting cells in the gastric mucosa producing a profuse flow of gastric juice with a high acidity but relatively low pepsin content.

H_1 receptor antagonists such as mepyramine, chlorcyclizine and the other standard antihistamine drugs antagonise both the excitant and depressant actions of histamine on cortical neurones, but they also antagonise the depressant effects of acetylcholine, noradrenaline and 5–HT. Thus the extent to which their central effects are due to antihistamine activity is uncertain.

A histamine-sensitive adenylate cyclase has been described in rat neocortex and hippocampus, with the pharmacological characteristics of an H_2 receptor. H_2 receptors are selectively blocked by cimetidine and ranitidine. These drugs can cause drowsiness and mental confusion in standard doses for treatment of peptic ulcer in patients with impairment of excretion due to renal disease. Intravenous, but not oral, cimetidine can produce a rise in plasma prolactin levels. It appears, therefore, that there are H_2 receptors within the human brain.

Inhibitory aminoacids

Gamma-aminobutyric acid (GABA) is restricted in its distribution to the central nervous system, and is present in larger amounts than any of the other aminoacids. It acts as a post-synaptic inhibitory transmitter in the cerebral and cerebellar cortex, while in the spinal cord it mediates presynaptic inhibition of afferent pathways. Inhibitors of GABA-transaminase, the enzyme that degrades GABA, have anticonvulsant activity. GABA mimetic drugs may mimic its effects within the nervous system. Some, such as muscimol, are true GABA mimetics that interact directly with GABA receptors. Others, such as baclofen, cause release of GABA from intracellular stores. The benzodiazepines (page 187) have a high affinity for specific receptors, stimulation of which facilitates the actions of GABA. The mechanism for this facilitation is uncertain but may involve: (a) displacement of an endogenous inhibitor of GABA receptor binding, so permitting more endogenous GABA to reach and bind receptors, or (b) modification of the coupling of GABA receptors to the chloride ion channel thus enhancing GABA ergic inhibition.

Glycine is found particularly in the nerve terminals of spinal interneurones, and probably acts as a post-synaptic inhibitory transmitter on motoneurones.

Taurine is found in several areas of rat brain. Iontophoretic application on to single central neurones depresses their activity, suggesting that it may have an inhibitory function. Taurine deficiency is associated with retinal degeneration in cats. Its role, if any, in the human brain and its disorders is not yet known.

Adenosine The central pharmacological effects of the xanthines (e.g. caffeine) are thought to involve adenosine receptors.

Excitatory aminoacids

Glutamic acid is the most important excitatory aminoacid in the central nervous system. It is released from the cerebral cortex when the reticular formation is stimulated electrically, and excites many different types of neurone, including cortical neurones and spinal motor neurones, when applied to them iontophoretically. Although both its isomers are pharmacologically active, the L isomer is reported to be more active than the D.

Aspartic acid, formed from glutamate by transmination with oxaloacetate, also has central excitatory activity.

Peptides

A large number of peptides have been isolated from nerve tissue and are known to be released from neurones. However the roles of most of them as neurotransmitters have not yet been confirmed (Table 1). They may be subdivided into three groups.

(a) The opioid peptides, enkephalins, endorphins and dynorphins bind to specific receptors within the brain. Met-enkephalin and leu-enkephalin are pentapeptides found in many areas of the brain. Met-enkephalin has the same aminoacid sequence as the acids 61–65 in the larger peptide β–endorphin which in turn is part of

Table 1   *Peptides that may have a transmitter role in the central nervous system*

Peptide	Localised within neurones	Action on neurones	Released from neurones	Mimics physiological stimulation of specific pathway
Opioid peptides	Yes	Inhibits	Yes	Not tested
Substance P	Yes	Excites	Yes	Yes
Angiotensin II	Yes	Excites?	Not tested	Not tested
Cholecystokinin and gastrin	Yes	Excite?	Yes	Not tested
Vasopressin and oxytocin	Yes	Inhibit	Yes	Not tested
Somatostatin	Yes	Inhibits	Yes	Not tested
Neurotensin	Yes	Excites	Not tested	Not tested
Thyrotrophin-releasing hormone	Yes	Inhibits	Yes	Not tested
Vasoactive intestinal peptide	Yes	Excites	Yes	Not tested

Based on Cooper *et al.*, *The Biochemical Basis of Neuropharmacology*, 4th edn, Oxford University Press, New York, 1982

17

the still larger β-lipotropin. β-endorphin is found in the brain but with a different distribution from the enkephalins, and is also found in the pituitary gland. Although enkephalins and endorphins have important functions in influencing behavioural responses to painful stimuli, they also appear to play a role in regulating secretion of some pituitary hormones, thermoregulation, eating, learning, sexual behaviour and the regulation of central cardiovascular control and respiration.

(b) Substance P, angiotensin II, and cholecystokinin, were originally described in relation to their action on the smooth muscle of blood vessels and viscera, but are now known to be present within the brain. Substance P is a small polypeptide of eleven aminoacids with neuronal localisation in areas related to pain appreciation, particularly cells of the posterior root ganglion projecting to the substantia gelatinosa of the spinal cord, the hypothalamus and thalamus. Although there is still controversy about its physiological role, there is evidence that while enkephalins are involved in suppression of pain, substance P appears to mediate its enhancement. Angiotensin II, an octapeptide, is also found in many areas of the brain, particularly in those thought to be related to pain. Cholecystokinin is found within the brain in the form of its octapeptide, particularly in the cerebral cortex, but its physiological role is not yet known.

The two very similar nonapeptides oxytocin and vasopressin, which have well-known peripheral effects on the uterus and kidney, are synthesised in the supraoptic and paraventricular nuclei and are stored in axons of neurones arising within them, from which they are released into the circulation. These neurones also project on to target cells in the mid brain and hippocampus, and may have a transmitter role in these areas. There is experimental evidence for behavioural actions of vasopressin and structural analogues. Subcutaneous administration to rats delays extinction of learned aversive or appetitive tasks. In man, administration by nasal spray has been claimed to enhance performance in short-term memory tests. The significance of these observations is under investigation.

(c) Somatostatin and neurotensin were identified in the hypo-thalamus during research on hypothalamic releasing factors for pituitary hormones. Somatostatin is a tetradecapeptide, 90 per cent of its brain content being found outside the hypothalamus, including the amygdala and posterior root ganglia. Neurotensin, a tridecapeptide, also occurs in other areas of the central nervous system as well as the hypothalamus. Their physiological function is still uncertain, although animal studies suggest that they are related to responsiveness to noxious stimuli.

In addition, other peptides such as thyrotropin-releasing hormone and vasoactive intestinal peptide have been identified in certain cell groups of the brain, and probably have a neurotransmitter role.

Prostaglandins

Prostaglandin was the name given by Von Euler in 1935 to a lipid substance derived from human seminal fluid which contracted smooth muscle. Substances with similar pharmacological activity were found in the seminal fluid of sheep, and in extracts of prostate and vesicular glands. Today the term 'prostaglandins' no longer refers to a single substance but to a large family of closely related long-chain unsaturated fatty acids, all derivatives of prostanoic acid.

Several prostaglandins, including E and F, are present in the mammalian central nervous system, and are released from the cerebral cortex into a perfusing fluid when peripheral nerves are stimulated. This release is depressed by drugs such as pentobarbitone and chlorpromazine. Some of these compounds have been studied with microinjection techniques and have excitant and inhibitory actions on various neurones in the brain stem. Their action is prolonged when compared with other transmitter substances such as acetylcholine and noradrenaline, and, although their presence in the brain and release on nerve stimulation suggests some function relating to transmission, it may be that this is more concerned with control or modulation of transmitter release or neuronal excitability than actual transmission.

Cyclic nucleotides

The neurotransmitters, or putative transmitters, that have so far been discussed may be considered as 'first' or 'primary' messengers. Stimulation of their specific cell surface receptors is thought to initiate a secondary event within the target cells, mediated by a 'second messenger', probably one of two cyclic nucleotides, cyclic AMP (cyclic 3^1, 5^1 adenosine monophosphate) (Figure 2) and cyclic GMP (cyclic 3^1, 5^1 guanosine monophosphate). Their rate of

19

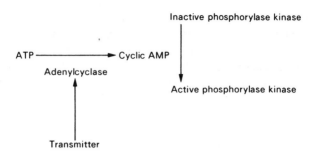

Figure 2 *Activation of cyclic AMP by a neurotransmitter mediated by the enzyme adenyl cyclase*

production is mediated by receptor stimulation through two enzymes, adenylate cyclase and guanylate cyclase respectively. Cyclic AMP appears to be activated in the central nervous system by NA, dopamine, histamine and substance P, and it is possible that the actions of 5–HT and prostaglandins may also be mediated through it. Cyclic GMP appears to be linked to muscarinic cholinergic receptors.

Increase in nucleotide production results in increased activation of protein kinase, to phosphorylate a protein substrate. This in turn leads to a change in ion permeability resulting in depolarisation or hyperpolarisation of the cell membrane.

Transmitter synthesis, release, uptake and metabolism

Although very little is known of the synthesis, release and metabolism of transmitters within the central nervous system, a considerable amount of information has been obtained in recent years about the handling of acetylcholine and noradrenaline at peripheral synapses, and it is probable that similar mechanisms apply centrally. For convenience, present knowledge regarding noradrenaline in sympathetic neurones will be discussed in more detail and, where appropriate, extrapolation from this to other transmitters such as acetylcholine, dopamine and 5–HT, will be made.

Noradrenaline is present in sympathetic nerve terminals in several stores or pools, being localised in terminal ramifications of the neurone which have a beaded, varicose appearance. Adrenergic neurones in the brain have a similar appearance. Approximately 40 per cent of the noradrenaline is free in the cytoplasm and the other 60 per cent is in intra-granular stores, called 'synaptic vesicles', where it is bound to protein and hence is relatively resistant to metabolising enzymatic activity. The release of noradrenaline from the vesicles into the synaptic cleft takes place by a process called exocytosis in which the vesicle membrane fuses with the cellular wall and the contents of the vesicle are extruded. The passage of the neurotransmitter-containing vesicles along the microtubules within the axon towards the pre-synaptic terminals is influenced by nerve impulses. It is carried in the opposite direction by active transport mechanisms from the extracellular space to the cytoplasm, and from the cytoplasm into the vesicles. Binding of noradrenaline to protein within the vesicles probably represents a separate active process in which adenosine triphosphate (ATP) is involved.

There are two sources of the noradrenaline in the vesicles and cytoplasm:

1 Local synthesis from phenylalanine
2 Uptake from the extracellular space of noradrenaline which may either have been released locally, or have come from distant sites such as the adrenal medulla, or have been administered exogenously.

When isotopically labelled noradrenaline is injected intravenously into animals it rapidly disappears from the circulation. About half of it is metabolised, while the rest is actively taken up by adrenergic fibres and can be demonstrated radiographically in the cytoplasm and granules. When a post-ganglionic sympathetic nerve is cut and allowed to degenerate, its ability to accumulate exogenous noradrenaline disappears.

An understanding of noradrenaline uptake is important from the point of view of its inactivation after it has acted at the receptor site, for its binding within the cell represents a way in which it can be inactivated and used again.

The enzymatic metabolism of noradrenaline is largely dependent on two groups of enzymes: monoamine oxidase (MAO) and catechol-O-methyltransferase (COMT).

Monoamine oxidase is widely distributed throughout the body; within the brain it is present in larger quantities in the hypothalamus than elsewhere. It is concerned with the metabolism of a wide variety of compounds, including noradrenaline, dopamine and 5–HT, and is located intracellularly in mitochondria at synaptic nerve endings, being partly responsible for regulating the cytoplasmic levels of these amines. It exists in at least two forms, A and B.

Catechol-O-methyltransferase is also widely distributed in brain tissue, and S-adenosylmethionine which is its cofactor is formed in the brain. Unlike MAO, it is responsible for the extracellular metabolism of noradrenaline, which has diffused passively through the cell membrane or that which is released by nerve stimulation or drugs, and of catecholamines released from the adrenal medulla.

The steps in the metabolic degradation of noradrenaline, dopamine and 5–HT are shown in the diagram.

It seems likely that when a nerve impulse arrives at the end of an adrenergic neurone, storage particles of bound noradrenaline, or

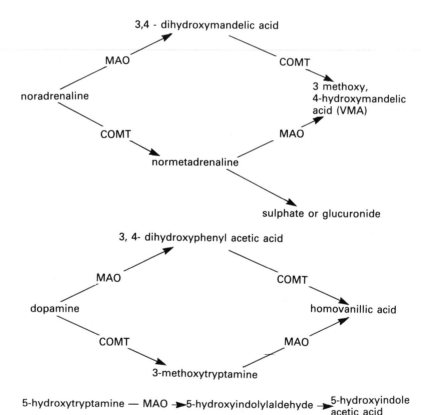

synaptic vesicles, fuse with the neuronal cell membrane under the influence of calcium ions which enter the cell, and then discharge their contents into the 'synaptic cleft' or extracellular space. The released noradrenaline stimulates receptors on the effector cell surface, and is then either taken up again into the pre-synaptic neurone, or is metabolised outside the cell by COMT, or is carried away by extracellular fluid.

The series of events which have been described for noradrenaline probably apply to other transmitters. 5–HT is synthesised within brain neurones from its precursor tryptophan and is metabolised by MAO. It is probably stored, and released in a similar manner to noradrenaline, and there appears to be a similar uptake process for this amine. Acetylcholine is synthesised from choline within brain neurones, and is rapidly destroyed on release by acetylcholinesterase. When acetylcholinesterase is inhibited there is some evidence of an uptake process for acetylcholine also.

Pre-synaptic inhibition and facilitation

There is good evidence that, as well as stimulatory receptors on the post-synaptic cell surface, the neurotransmitter stimulates receptors on the pre-synaptic membrane (Figure 3). This usually functions as a negative feedback mechanism, to regulate its further release. In the case of noradrenergic fibres, it is probable that stimulation of pre-synaptic alpha-2 receptors (see page 26) mediates a decrease in noradrenaline release while pre-synaptic beta-receptor stimulation mediates facilitation of noradrenaline release. Blockade of pre-synaptic alpha receptors therefore leads to an increase, and of beta receptors a decrease, in transmitter release. It is probable that there are pre-synaptic receptors for a variety of substances on noradrenergic, dopaminergic, cholinergic and 5–HT neurones, including GABA, peptides and prostaglandins, which are therefore said to *modulate* release of these transmitters.

Receptors

Neurohumoral agents and transmitters such as those which have been described earlier in this chapter are composed, like other drugs, of molecules. The result of their action on post-synaptic cells must eventually be explained in terms of an interaction of these molecules, or parts of them, with specific molecules on the post-

23

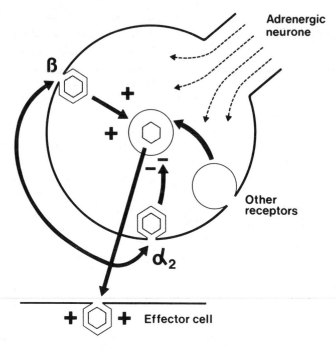

Figure 3 *Diagrammatic representation of adrenergic nerve ending and presynaptic and postsynaptic receptors. Presynaptic receptors may facilitate (β) or inhibit (α2) transmitter release*

synaptic cell membrane. The latter are called the 'specific receptors' for the transmitter or drug with respect to the particular effect. The term 'receptor' is usually limited to drug–cell or transmitter–cell combinations that initiate a sequence of specific effects. Other drug–cell or transmitter–cell interactions that do not initiate these specific effects, such as binding of drugs to plasma, binding of neurotransmitter to cell protein and to enzymes for transport, storage and biotransformation, are referred to in other terms such as 'secondary receptors', 'storage sites' or 'drug acceptors'.

Little is known of the chemistry of receptor substances in the central nervous system. It is possible to make certain tentative suggestions on their nature, however, on the basis of what is known about their counterparts in the peripheral autonomic system. Much of our knowledge of these has been gained from studies using specific receptor-blocking drugs, but often these drugs do not pass readily into the brain from the vascular system and so their usefulness in studying central receptors is limited.

Cholinergic receptors

The peripheral autonomic effects of acetylcholine are similar to those produced by the alkaloid muscarine and thus are known as its 'muscarinic actions', as distinct from its actions on ganglia and neuromuscular junctions which resemble those of nicotine, the so-called 'nicotinic' actions. Microinjection of acetylcholine into the brain and spinal cord, and studies in whole animals and isolated tissues with the tremor-producing compound oxotremorine, suggest that central cholinergic receptors are predominantly muscarinic and are blocked by compounds which block muscarinic receptors such as atropine and hyoscine. However, in several areas of the brain and spinal cord there is evidence of nicotinic receptors, or of receptors which appear to be intermediate between the nicotinic and muscarinic type.

The synthesis of the selective antimuscarinic drug pirenzepine has led to the subdivision of muscarine receptors into the M_1 subtype with a high affinity for pirenzepine and M_2 receptors with a low affinity for it. Pirenzepine has been shown to antagonise certain memory processes in rats, and it has been suggested that selective M_1 receptor agonists might be used to alleviate the cholinergic deficit and, perhaps, the memory impairment in Alzheimer's disease.

Adrenergic receptors (adrenoceptors)

In 1948, Ahlquist suggested that the effects of adrenaline at peripheral sympathetic sites could be divided into two groups with two types of receptor, alpha and beta. These were originally called 'excitatory' and 'inhibitory' receptors, respectively, because of their general tendency to produce excitation or inhibition when stimulated, but as there are important exceptions to this in both groups, it is better to refer to them only as alpha and beta receptors. Noradrenaline has predominantly alpha-adrenergic activity, the most important in man being vasoconstriction of arterioles in the skin and splanchnic area, producing a rise in systemic blood pressure, dilatation of the pupil and relaxation of the gut. The beta actions are mimicked by the synthetic sympathomimetic drug isoprenaline and include acceleration of the heart, dilatation of arterioles supplying skeletal muscles, bronchial relaxation and relaxation of the uterus. Drugs which selectively block alpha actions are known as adrenergic alpha-2 receptor blocking drugs and include phenoxybenzamine, phentolamine, thymoxamine and tolazoline. The adrenergic beta receptor sites may be blocked selectively by a variety of related drugs including propranolol, oxprenolol, pindolol, alprenolol and sotalol. No sympathomimetic drug yet available has pure alpha or beta stimulating actions. When the alpha receptor effects of noradrenaline are blocked, for example by thymoxamine, its weaker beta receptor actions are seen, and even the potent beta receptor agonist compound, isoprenaline, can be shown to have weak alpha stimulating properties when its beta receptor actions are blocked with propranolol. Pre-synaptic receptors (page 23) appear to be of both alpha and beta type; stimulation of the alpha (α_2) receptors inhibits further noradrenaline release, while pre-synaptic beta receptor stimulation facilitates it. Pre-synaptic alpha receptor blockade facilitates, and beta receptor blockade inhibits, noradrenaline release.

Although the alpha and beta receptor actions appear to be so different, it is probable that the actual receptor substance is the same, namely adenylcyclase. This enzyme catalyses the conversion of ATP to cyclic AMP, and is widely distributed in a large number of animal tissues.

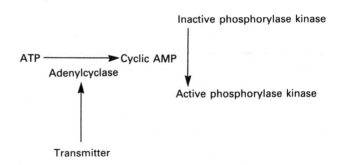

Catecholamines, such as adrenaline, noradrenaline and isoprenaline, have a central stimulating action, which gives rise to anxiety and restlessness; this stimulating action is probably due, at least in part, to stimulation of central receptors, through the same adenylcyclase-receptor mechanism as in the periphery.

Dopaminergic receptors

There are two basic types of dopamine (DA) receptors; one being linked to an adenylate cyclase – cyclic AMP mechanism in a fashion similar to that obtaining for the noradrenergic receptors. This adenylate cyclase linked receptor is usually referred to as the D_1 receptor; the other, non-adenylate cyclase linked receptor being called a D_2 receptor.

There are certain pharmacological differences between D_1 and D_2 receptors. D_1 receptors, for example, are more sensitive to the agonist effects of DA itself than are D_2; the same is true of apomorphine, in fact apomorphine appears to act as an antagonist rather than an agonist at D_1 receptors. As far as DA receptor blocking drugs are concerned, the butyrophenones, such as haloperiedol, are more potent antagonists of D_2 receptors than of D_1, and sulpiride, the substituted benzamide compound, acts almost exclusively on D_2 receptors. However, other categories of antipsychotic drugs such as the phenothiazines and the thioxanthines, do not display such differential activity.

Anatomically, the post-synaptic DA receptors within the striatum mediating neurotransmission from the nigro-striatal tract are largely D_1 receptors, whereas those in the pituitary regulating the DA mediated inhibition of prolactin release are D_2. Pre-synaptic autoreceptors are also thought to be largely D_2 receptors.

It is as yet unknown which type of DA receptor mechanism is involved in the pathogenesis of schizophrenia (see chapter 6) although the reports that the relatively specific D_2 receptor antagonist sulpiride is effective in this condition (see page 116) suggest that D_2 receptors are involved.

5-hydroxytryptamine receptors

There appears to be at least three types of receptor for 5HT in the body. The older classification of D and M receptors has been replaced by $5HT_1$, $5HT_2$ and $5HT_3$. The $5HT_1$ receptors are limited to adenylate cyclase. Most peripheral $5HT_1$ receptors in platelets and smooth muscle appear to be of the $5HT_2$ type. All three receptor types have been identified in the brain.

GABA receptors

See page 16.

Antidepressant binding sites

Autoradiographic studies have demonstrated a wide distribution of binding sites in the brain for imipramine and desipramine. These sites seem to be distinct from 5–HT and catecholamine binding sites, and their significance, if any, in the pathogenesis and treatment of psychiatric illness is not yet clear.

Calcium-antagonist receptors

Calcium ions regulate many cellular functions, including neurotransmitter secretion by neurones. Levels of calcium in cytoplasm are maintained through regulation of its entry into the cell. Stimulation of the cell produces either opening of calcium channels in the cell membrane or release of intracellular calcium stores. Calcium antagonist drugs interfere with the entry of calcium into cells through voltage-sensitive channels, but do not significantly affect its intracellular storage. Biophysical studies suggest that calcium antagonists do not act by physically blocking membrane pores through which calcium ions pass, but that they bind to receptors on the cell membrane, stimulation of which results in inhibition of calcium transport.

Binding sites for calcium antagonists have been found in various regions of the brain including the hippocampus and substantia nigra, areas clearly associated with synaptic transmission and not with blood vessels. Studies with dihydropyridine calcium antagonists such as nifedipine and nitrendipine have shown that they block calcium-mediated release of 5–HT from brain slices.

It is possible that the action of some neuroleptic drugs involves calcium antagonism. Studies with diphenylbutylpiperidines, the group of drugs to which pimozide and fluspirilene belong, have shown that they are as potent antagonists of calcium entry sites as of dopamine D_2 receptors.

Specificity of neuronal transmitter release and receptor response

Microinjection techniques have shown that neurones in many areas of the brain respond to a variety of neurotransmitters, both excitatory and inhibitory. There is also evidence that neurones may secrete more than one transmitter. In particular, cotransmission of 'modulatory' peptides and prostaglandins (pages 17–19) may be the rule rather than the exception.

Mechanisms of the action of psychotropic drugs

From this brief review of the probable pharmacological basis of central nervous transmission, it is evident that a drug may interfere with central nervous function in a variety of ways (see Figure 4):

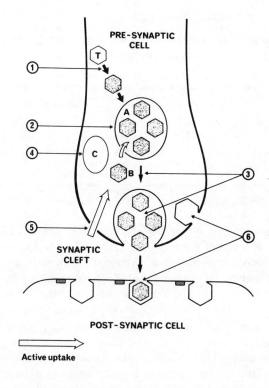

Figure 4   *Diagrammatic representation of a central monoaminergic synapse showing possible sites of drug action*
A, granular pool of monoamine. B, cytoplasmic pool of monoamine. C, monoamine oxidase. T, precursor of monoamines (tyrosine, tryptophan, etc.). 1–6 sites of drug action as described in the text.

GENERAL PRINCIPLES

(a) Inhibition of synthesis of transmitter substances
(b) Production of 'false transmitter'
(c) Increased precursor load
(d) Depletion of transmitter from neurones
(e) Inhibition of release of transmitter
(f) Release of transmitter from neurones on to receptor
(g) Monoamine oxidase inhibition
(h) Uptake inhibition
(i) Receptor stimulation, pre-synaptic and post-synaptic
(j) Receptor blockade, pre-synaptic and post-synaptic
(k) Receptor modulation

Inhibition of transmitter synthesis (site 1)

Several compounds are known to block the synthesis of one or more transmitters in animals, but little is known of their effects in man.

The synthesis of noradrenaline in man is inhibited by at least two substances which are used clinically. Alpha-methylparatyrosine inhibits the conversion of tyrosine to dopa by the enzyme tyrosine hydroxylase, which is the rate-limiting step in noradrenaline biosynthesis. This reduces tissue levels of noradrenaline, but 5–HT levels remain unchanged. When used clinically in the management of patients with phaeochromocytoma, alpha-methylparatyrosine tends to produce sedation, while mild anxiety and insomnia often appear after sudden withdrawal of the drug.

Alpha-methyldopa is an antihypertensive agent which also reduces tissue levels of noradrenaline. This effect is due, in part, to inhibition of dopa decarboxylase, interfering with the conversion of dopa to dopamine. The enzyme is also concerned in the production of dopamine, histamine and 5–HT, and levels of these transmitters in tissues such as the brain and heart are reduced at the same time as noradrenaline. Sedation occurs in almost all patients treated with methyldopa, but tends to disappear as treatment continues.

The biosynthesis of 5–HT in the brain is inhibited by p-chlorophenylalanine which blocks tryptophan hydroxylase activity, the rate-limiting enzyme for 5–HT synthesis. Its behavioural effects are not marked, and administration of large doses to experimental animals does not appear to produce consistent stimulant or inhibiting effects. However, pre-treatment with p-chlorophenylalanine interferes with the characteristic pharmacological effects of other drugs, such as LSD, which interact with 5–HT mechanisms in the brain.

Production of false neurotransmitter (site 1)

A drug may be taken up into a nerve cell and metabolised so that it replaces the normal transmitter and is later released on nerve stimulation or by other drugs. The effects of such drugs·on the receptors may either be similar to or different from those of the physiological transmitter substances. There is evidence that alpha-methylnoradrenaline stimulates central alpha adrenergic receptors in the nucleus of the tractus solitarius or in the vasomotor centre, which mediate reduction in sympathetic outflow, and so lower blood pressure.

The antihypertensive drug alpha-methyldopa already referred to in the previous section is thought to act in part by competing with dopa for decarboxylation by dopa decarboxylase so that the following biosynthesis occurs:

Alpha-methyldopa ⟶ Alpha-methyldopamine ⟶
Alpha-methylnoradrenaline

Alpha-methylnoradrenaline, therefore, replaces noradrenaline in equimolar concentrations in adrenergic neurones and may be released by nerve impulses as a false transmitter with noradrenaline (the physiological transmitter). Alpha-methylnoradrenaline appears to be as potent, if not more so, as an agonist at central alpha adrenoceptors in nuclei in the floor of the fourth ventricle, stimulation of which results in a decrease in sympathetic outflow leading to a fall in blood pressure.

There is considerable evidence that amphetamine, after releasing noradrenaline, is metabolised in nervous tissue to p-hydroxy-norephedrine. This compound, which may then replace nor-adrenaline in adrenergic neurones, has less receptor stimulant activity than noradrenaline or alpha-methylnoradrenaline. The formation of p-hydroxynorephedrine with its lesser stimulant action may thus account in part for the tolerance which develops to the central and peripheral effects of amphetamine.

After inhibition of monoamine oxidase, endogenous tyramine, which is normally metabolised by this enzyme, accumulates in neural tissue together with its hydroxylated derivative octopamine. The latter accumulates in nerve endings in the brain, as well as peripherally, and is released by nerve stimulation to act as a false transmitter in competition with noradrenaline. The extent to which any of the behavioural changes, induced by monoamine oxidase inhibition, are due to the effects of octopamine is not yet known.

Increased precursor load (site 1)

Administration to an animal or man of a precursor of a neurotransmitter substance may lead to increased synthesis of the transmitter, provided that rate-limiting steps in the synthetic pathway are not already fully loaded. Thus, administration of levodopa orally or parenterally leads to an increase of dopamine in the basal ganglia and of noradrenaline in some other tissues.

Tryptophan administered orally is hydroxylated to form 5–hydroxytryptophan which in turn is decarboxylated to 5–hydroxytryptamine.

$$\text{tryptophan} \xrightarrow[\text{hydroxylase}]{\text{tryptophan}} \text{5-hydroxytryptophan} \xrightarrow[\text{5-hydroxytryptamine}]{\text{decarboxylase}}$$

Similarly histidine is the precursor of histamine and is readily converted to it by the enzyme histidine decarboxylase.

Possible clinical implications of the use of some of these precursors will be described in later chapters.

Depletion of transmitter from neurones (site 2)

Reserpine is an alkaloid obtained from the roots of *Rauwolfia serpentina*, a climbing shrub indigenous to India and neighbouring countries. More than twenty alkaloids can be extracted from this plant with a wide variety of pharmacological actions, the most important of which is the depletion of tissue stores of noradrenaline, adrenaline, dopamine, 5–HT and histamine, particularly in the brain. This depletion probably involves inhibited binding of these monoamines in the intracytoplasmic granular stores so that they are more vulnerable to monoamine oxidase activity. The amine-depleting action results in two important therapeutic effects, namely the calming of manic and schizophrenic patients, and an antihypertensive effect in patients with hypertension. These therapeutic actions may easily become serious unwanted effects, however, for further amine depletion can itself produce severe depression (see chapter 7). Whether this is due to specific depletion of either noradrenaline or 5–HT, or of both together, is not yet certain. Its dopamine-depleting effects result in parkinsonism which may be accompanied by choreoathetosis and cerebellar ataxia.

Alpha-methyldopa is another compound which produces depletion of noradrenaline, dopamine, 5–HT and histamine from the brain. At least two mechanisms for this have already been described, namely inhibition of synthesis, and replacement of the physiological transmitter by a 'false' one. This depletion probably accounts for the sedation and depression which commonly occur with its use, and for the parkinsonism which may be seen with high doses over long periods of time.

Inhibition of release of transmitter (site 3)

Some antihypertensive drugs such as bethanidine, debrisoquine and guanethidine are thought to interfere with peripheral sympathetic nerve activity by preventing release of noradrenaline from the nerve ending. They do not have significant behavioural effects in antihypertensive doses, possibly because of their failure to penetrate the brain. It is unlikely that any psychotropic drugs now in use act predominantly by this mechanism.

Release of transmitter from neurone on to receptor (site 3)

Sympathomimetic amines, which mimic the effects of sympathetic stimulation, may be broadly divided into two groups (see Table 2). The first group of catecholamines comprising adrenaline, noradrenaline, isoprenaline and dopamine, together with some other amines such as phenylephrine, depend mainly for their effects on direct stimulation of adrenergic receptors. The second group depend mainly for their effects on their ability to be taken up into the sympathetic nerve terminal and then to release noradrenaline from the synaptic vesicles in the nerve ending on to the receptor. They are, therefore, called 'indirectly acting' sympathomimetic compounds. This distribution is easily demonstrated in the peripheral autonomic system, for example in the eye, where depletion of noradrenaline by sympathectomy leads to abolition of the mydriatic effects of ephedrine, tyramine, amphetamine and

Table 2 *Classification of sympathomimetic amines into predominant direct and indirect activity*

Directly acting	Adrenaline
	Noradrenaline
	Dopamine
	Isoprenaline
	Salbutamol
	Phenylephrine
	Methoxamine
Indirectly acting	Amphetamine
	Ephedrine
	Hydroxyamphetamine
	Phenmetrazine
	Tyramine

phenmetrazine while the effects of phenylephrine and adrenaline persist.

It is probable that the central actions of amphetamine, phenmetrazine and other indirectly acting amines also depend on the liberation of noradrenaline and dopamine from central adrenergic and dopaminergic neurones. Animal experiments have shown that the central stimulant action of dexamphetamine is almost completely blocked by pre-treatment with reserpine, and by compounds which inhibit noradrenaline and dopamine synthesis. Its activity is restored, however, by very small doses of dopa which have no effects in the normal animal. The relative importance of dopamine and noradrenaline in mediating various components of the central effects of amphetamine is still not certain. The problem is complicated by the possible 'false transmitter' role of metabolites of amphetamine such as p-hydroxynorephedrine, already described.

It may well be that other centrally acting drugs act in part or whole by releasing one or more transmitter substances from central neurones.

Monoamine oxidase inhibition (site 4)

Inhibition of the action of the intracellular enzyme monoamine oxidase (MAO) leads to an accumulation within the nerve of monoamines such as noradrenaline, dopamine, 5–HT and histamine. This occurs both peripherally and centrally. Monoamine oxidase is in fact a general term for a series of more specific enzymes which deal with the individual monoamines, but MAO inhibitors tend to inhibit the whole family of enzymes, and thus lead to an increase in all the amines. A large number of drugs inhibit MAO to a limited extent, including cocaine and amphetamine, but their main actions do not appear to depend on this property. In the case of other compounds, including the hydrazine derivatives iproniazid and phenelzine and the amphetamine derivative tranylcypromine, their pharmacological actions probably do depend on MAO inhibition. The hydrazine group produce a long-lasting inhibition by an irreversible, non-competitive inhibition of the enzyme *in vitro* and *in vivo*. In contrast, the harmala alkaloids, harmine and harmaline, produce a short-lasting, reversible competitive inhibition of the enzyme.

The MAO enzyme appears to exist in two forms. MAO-A includes 5–HT and NA among its preferential substrates. MAO-B includes dopamine among its preferential substrates. Tyramine is a substrate for both forms.

Most MAO inhibitors such as phenelzine are non-selective. Clorgyline is a selective inhibitor of MAO-A, while selegiline (see page 154) is a selective inhibitor of MAO-B, and has already found therapeutic uses in Parkinson's disease and narcolepsy.

Inhibition of MAO enhances the elevation of brain catecholamine and 5–HT concentrations and the central stimulation produced by precursors of these transmitters. It also reverses the central depression and amine-depleting effects of reserpine, and enhances the central stimulant effects of drugs such as amphetamine which release central stores of noradrenaline.

Uptake inhibition (site 5)

Uptake of noradrenaline into the adrenergic nerve terminals represents a major route of its inactivation, and it is probable that a similar mechanism operates with other transmitter substances including dopamine and 5–HT. Inhibition of this uptake would lead to an increase in the activity of transmitter at the receptor site.

A large number of drugs have been shown to interfere with noradrenaline uptake, including many with actions on the central nervous system. Among these are the central stimulant compounds amphetamine and cocaine, the antidepressant drugs imipramine and tranylcypromine, and the tranquillising drugs chlorpromazine and reserpine. Because of the wide spectrum of clinical effects shown by drugs which possess this action it is probable that, in the case of most of these compounds, inhibition of uptake, though an interesting pharmacological phenomenon, does not contribute to the primary clinical effect. In the case of the dibenzazepine drugs, however, such as imipramine, it is probable that inhibition of uptake with increase of transmitter at the receptor site plays an important role in its main therapeutic action. Furthermore, it has been suggested that at least part of the central action of the phenothiazine compounds, such as chlorpromazine, is the result of partial blockage of noradrenaline uptake at sites where the latter acts as an inhibitory transmitter, so leading to a potentiation of its inhibiting effects.

It might be argued that facilitation of uptake with increase of intraneuronal breakdown of noradrenaline by MAO could lead to a decrease in the concentration of transmitter at central receptor sites. This, in fact, is one of the suggested modes of action for lithium salts in the prophylaxis of manic depressive psychosis (see chapter 7).

While the inhibition or facilitation of monoamine uptake into animal brain slices can be readily demonstrated, studies in man are largely limited to the use of changes in noradrenaline or tyramine pressor effects as a measure of noradrenaline reuptake, and to changes in platelet dopamine and 5–HT uptake.

Under carefully controlled conditions, the human platelet actively takes up 5–HT and noradrenaline, probably through the same uptake process. Monoamine reuptake-inhibiting drugs such as imipramine inhibit this uptake process; some, such as clomipramine, inhibit 5–HT uptake selectively. Platelets from patients with endogenous depression show reduced uptake of 5–HT and dopamine compared with normal controls, but the mechanism of this is not clear. Studies in animals have shown that 5–HT uptake in rat platelets and brain cells is inhibited by treatment with ACTH or dexamethasone. Endogenous depression is associated with increased plasma cortisol levels, and the diminished platelet uptake of monoamines may be due to this rather than a primary defect associated with the condition.

Receptor stimulation (site 6)

Some compounds may exert their central effects by a direct stimulation of central post-synaptic receptors. Apomorphine, bromocriptine, lisuride and piribedil are thought to stimulate dopamine receptors, and the tremor-producing compound, oxotremorine, may stimulate central cholinergic receptors. The antihypertensive drug clonidine is thought to reduce sympathetic outflow by stimulating central pre-synaptic alpha adrenoceptors in nuclei in the flow of the fourth ventricle.

Pre-synaptic beta receptor stimulation with salbutamol may enhance transmitter release and account for its claimed anti-depressant effects (page 156).

Receptor blockade (site 6)

Many drugs are known to block specifically adrenergic, cholinergic and 5–HT receptors in the peripheral autonomic system, and it is probable that the central actions of some compounds are due to a similar mechanism. For example, the sedating effects of hyoscine may well be due to central cholinergic receptor blockade. It is probable also that phenothiazine drugs, such as chlorpromazine, owe the major part of their central effects to a dopamine receptor-blocking action, and the same may be true of the butyrophenones such as haloperidol. It is tempting to apply similar reasoning to the antihistamine compounds by suggesting that their central effects are due to histamine-receptor blockade in the brain.

Pre-synaptic alpha adrenoceptor blockade produces an increase in noradrenaline release from noradrenergic neurones, and it is probable that the antidepressive drug mianserin acts in this way to increase synaptic monoamine concentrations.

It is evident that there are several different ways in which a compound may produce central nervous effects when considered in terms of its interactions with neuronal processes at the transmitter level. Many compounds may have several different actions. For example, chlorpromazine has been shown in different experimental procedures to influence the release of noradrenaline, to affect its uptake into the neurone, and to block dopaminergic receptors. It is difficult to be certain which, if any, is the most significant. Similarly, the MAO inhibitors have a marked effect on the uptake, as well as the breakdown, of noradrenaline, and it is uncertain on which of these two actions their central stimulant effects depend.

Another example is that of propranolol, the beta adrenoceptor blocking drug which in low plasma concentrations of about

100 ng/ml acts predominantly by blocking beta receptors, but in higher concentrations of 1000 ng/ml and above, which are reached with the doses used in antipsychotic studies, probably has local anaesthetic, membrane stabilising and 5–HT inhibiting actions. Furthermore, the foregoing discussion has centred around the acute effects of drugs on the synthesis, release and uptake of transmitter substances and on receptor activity. Other factors, however, may be important:

1 *Regional variations in the site of action* For example, phenothiazines are thought to act primarily in the brain stem region, and benzodiazepines in the limbic system, while barbiturates probably act in a more diffuse and non-specific manner through the cortex and subcortical structures.

2 *Pre-synaptic inhibition and facilitation* See page 23.

3 *Longer-term changes in monoamine and receptor activity* Feedback mechanisms on the rate of transmitter synthesis and in receptor activity are known to occur in response to the acute changes produced by drugs which have been described. In particular, post-synaptic receptor blockade tends to be followed by increased transmitter synthesis and release on one hand, together with 'up-regulation', that is an increase in the number, of receptors on the post-synaptic membrane. Conversely, an increase in synaptic transmitter concentration or receptor stimulation is followed by 'down-regulation', or a decrease in number, of receptors on the post-synaptic membrane. Recent evidence suggests that up- or down-regulation in one receptor population may be associated with similar changes in other receptor populations, a so-called 'heterologous regulation'. For example, up-regulation of beta receptors by propranalol has been shown to increase responsiveness to prostacyclin (PGI_2).

In association with these changes in receptor density, longer-term changes occur in the intracellular concentration of cyclic nucleotides. All these receptor and intracellular events may have important implications in terms of clinical responses to drugs.

4 *Membrane and intracellular processes* (other than those already discussed). Compounds may interfere with neuronal cell membrane activity and ion transport, so reducing the ability of the

transmitter substance to trigger off impulses in the post-synaptic cell. Other drugs may interfere with energy-releasing enzyme systems, so producing their effects beyond the receptor. Drugs which interfere with transmitter mechanisms may also affect these other, less well-defined factors, and so their actual mode of action is even more difficult to define.

Suggestions for further reading

BURROWS, G. D., and NERRY, J. S., *Advances in Human Psychoparmacology*, vol. 1, Jai Press, Connecticut, 1980.

CHAN, M., and LEE, P. H. K., 'Serotonin uptake and imipramine binding in rat platelets after chronic dexamethasone and amitriptyline treatment', *Pharmacological Research Communications*, vol. 17, 1985, pp. 619–32.

COOPER, J. R., BLOOM, F. E., and ROTH, R. H., *The Biochemical Basis of Neuropharmacology*, 4th edn, Oxford University Press, New York, 1982.

CORN, T. H., and CHECKLEY, S. A., 'The effects of desipramine treatment upon central adrenoceptor function in depressed patients and normal subjects', in *Clinical and Pharmacological Studies in Psychiatric Disorders*, ed. Burrows, G. D., Norman, T. A., and Dennerstein, L., John Libbey, Paris, 1985, pp. 8–16.

CUELLO, A. C., POLAK, J. M., and PEARSE, A. G. E., 'Substance P: a naturally occurring transmitter in human spinal cord', *Lancet*, vol. 2, 1976, p. 1054.

DAVIES, D. A., and REID, J. L., *Central Action of Drugs in Blood Pressure Regulation*, Pitman Medical, Tunbridge Wells, 1976.

ESSMAN, W. B., *Neurotransmitters, Receptors and Drug Action*, MTP, Lancaster, 1980.

GRAHAME-SMITH, D. G., and ORR, M. W., 'Clinical psychopharmacology', in *Recent Advances in Clinical Pharmacology*, vol. 1, ed. P. Turner and D. G. Shand, Churchill Livingstone, Edinburgh, 1978.

HOLLENBERG, M. D., 'Examples of homospecific and heterospecific receptor regulation', *Trends in Pharmacological Science*, vol. 6, 1985, pp. 242–5.

HORNYKIEWICZ, O., 'Parkinson's disease and its chemotherapy', *Biochemical Pharmacology*, vol. 24, 1975, pp. 1061–5.

IVERSEN, L. L., IVERSEN, S. D., and SNYDER, S. H., *Biogenic Amine Receptors* (Handbook of Psychopharmacology, vol. 6), Plenum Press, New York, 1975.

JOHNSON, A. M., LOEW, D. M., and VIGOURET, J. M., 'Stimulant properties of bromocriptine on central dopamine receptors in comparison to apomorphine, (+) amphetamine and l-dopa', *British Journal of Pharmacology*, vol. 56, 1976, pp. 59–68.

KALSNER, S., *Trends in Autonomic Pharmacology*, vol. 3, Taylor & Francis, London, 1985.

KEBABIAN, J. W., and CALNE, D. B., 'Multiple receptors for dopamine', *Nature*, vol. 277, 1979, pp. 93–6.

LEVY, A., HELDMAN, E., VOGEL, Z., and GUTMAN, Y., 'Endogenous peptides and centrally acting drugs', *Progress in Biochemical Pharmacology*, vol. 16, Karger, Basel, 1980.

LIMA, D. A., and TURNER, P., 'Beta-blocking drugs increase responsiveness to prostacyclin in hypertensive patients', *Lancet*, vol. 2, 1982, p. 444.

SCHACHTER, M., 'Enkephalins and endorphins', *British Journal of Hospital Medicine*, vol. 25, 1981, pp. 128–36.

SLATER, P., 'Antidepressant binding sites in brain', *Clinical Science*, vol. 67, 1984, pp. 369–73.

SNYDER, S. H., and REYNOLDS, I. J., 'Calcium-antagonist drugs', *New England Journal of Medicine*, vol. 313, 1985, pp. 995–1002.

SWEET, W. H., 'Neuropeptides and monoaminergic neurotransmitters: their relation to pain', *Journal of the Royal Society of Medicine*, vol. 73, 1980, pp. 482–91.

VETULANI, J., and SULSER, F., 'Action of various antidepressant treatments reduces reactivity of noradrenergic cyclic AMP-generating system in limbic forebrain', *Nature*, vol. 257, 1975, pp. 495–6.

Factors influencing the action of psychotropic drugs   3

It is a fact of clinical experience that there is considerable variation from patient to patient in the response to a fixed dose of almost any drug. Such variation is at least partly due to the fact that the blood level of a drug following a given dose can vary by more than tenfold from one patient to another. It is not surprising, therefore, that in any patient population a given dose of a drug may produce a satisfactory therapeutic response in some, absence of effect in others, and evidence of intoxication in a further group. A number of factors are responsible for this phenomenon, apart from the obvious one of failure to take the prescribed dose of the drug (see chapter 5). The rate of absorption of the drug, its distribution throughout the body, its binding to plasma proteins and to tissues, its rate and routes of metabolism and excretion, all influence its concentration at the site of action and hence its clinical effects. Pharmacokinetics is the name given to study of these aspects of pharmacology, and rational prescribing depends on an understanding of pharmacokinetic principles.

Drug absorption

Following oral administration, a drug has to cross the bowel wall somewhere along its length to enter the circulation. Substances cross the gut mucosa in one or more of the following ways:

1 passive diffusion, which depends upon the concentration gradient
2 active transport against a concentration gradient by an energy-consuming mechanism
3 filtration through pores
4 pinocytosis, by which small particles are engulfed by mucosal cells

41

The first mechanism, passive diffusion, is the most important for drug absorption, and is influenced by several different factors:

A *The chemical nature of the drug* Most commonly used drugs are either weak acids (e.g. aspirin, barbiturates) or weak bases (e.g. amphetamine, tricyclic antidepressant drugs of the monoamine reuptake inhibitor type) (MARI), and these exist in two forms in solution, namely, as undissociated molecules and as ions. The equilibrium between these two forms is determined by (i) the pH of the surrounding medium, and (ii) the pK value of the drug. At a pH equal to the pKa the drug is 50 per cent ionised. At a low pH, for example in the stomach, a weakly acidic drug is mainly in its undissociated form whereas a weakly basic drug will be largely ionised. The reverse applies in an alkaline medium such as occurs in the small bowel.

In general, the undissociated molecules are more lipid soluble than the ionised species, and are thus more readily absorbed across the complex lipid membrane which is the gut mucosa. An alkaline medium, therefore, favours absorption of the weakly basic drugs.

B *Formulation* When a drug is prescribed the patient actually receives a medicine. The active substance may represent only a small proportion of the total weight of an oral solid dosage form such as a tablet or capsule. In recent years it has become increasingly realised that the other constituents of dosage forms are not necessarily inert but may facilitate or hinder a drug's absorption. Among the important factors involved in the production of tablets and capsules which may influence a drug's absorption are:

(i) Particle size of the drug. It was a change in particle size that produced the marked change in bioavailability of digoxin in Britain in the early 1970s.
(ii) Diluents, such as lactose or calcium sulphate which are used to increase bulk. A change in diluent led to an outbreak of phenytoin intoxication in Australia.
(iii) Granulating and binding agents, such as tragacanth, syrup or bentonite which assist aggregation of the powder into granules in order to permit compression into tablets.
(iv) Lubricants, such as talc, prevent granule adherence to the tableting machines.

(v) Disintegrating agents such as starch and cocoa butter are incorporated to produce rapid tablet disintegration in the gastrointestinal tract.

(vi) Coating materials such as sugar or the gelatin envelopes of capsules may prevent breakdown before the preparation reaches the stomach.

(vii) Special formulations employ complex pharmaceutical processes to control the rates of disintegration and dissolution and so to regulate the rate of a drug's absorption, for example in sustained release formulations.

C   *Gastric emptying and gut motility*   Most drugs are absorbed from the upper part of the small bowel, and drugs which delay gastric emptying, particularly those with anticholinergic activity such as amitriptyline or imipramine, can delay their own absorption and that of other drugs. Metoclopramide, which increases the rate of gastric emptying, may produce more rapid absorption of another drug given at the same time.

D   *Bowel wall and liver enzymes*   Unless a drug is absorbed directly into the systemic circulation, as from sublingual or rectal administration, it has to pass through the liver in the portal circulation. Furthermore, the gut mucosa also possesses some drug metabolising activity. Thus, when the indirectly acting sympatho-mimetic amines ephedrine or tyramine are ingested orally they are normally metabolised by the enzyme monoamine oxidase in the gut wall and liver. This enzyme is inhibited by monoamine oxidase inhibitors, allowing the passage of these substances into the systemic circulation (see page 155). Hepatic enzyme induction, on the other hand, can lead to increased metabolism of drugs in their passages through the liver (see page 49).

Distribution and protein binding

The lipid solubility of a drug not only influences its rate of absorption across the gut mucosa, but also its distribution throughout the body. A strongly basic drug such as the ganglion blocking drug hexamethonium is poorly absorbed from the gut, and when given parenterally, remains largely in the extracellular fluid. The blood–brain barrier consists of the vascular wall of the cerebral circulation and the tissue in contact with it. This is predominantly a lipid membrane which behaves very much like the gut wall as far as passive diffusion is concerned. Therefore, drugs which are well absorbed from the gut are usually able easily to enter the brain, provided they are not extensively protein-bound, for it is the unbound portion of the drug which is available to cross the lipid membrane. This presupposes, of course, that the drug is not completely metabolised as it passes through the liver into one or more compounds which are less lipid soluble and so less able to cross into the brain. A high degree of lipid solubility is a characteristic of centrally acting drugs, including anaesthetic agents both volatile and non-volatile such as thiopentone. These drugs, however, for the same reason, can easily cross the placenta to the foetal circulation, and it was a centrally acting drug (thalidomide) which produced such tragic teratogenic effects.

Most drugs are bound, to a greater or less degree, to plasma and tissue proteins. The extent of binding is important, as it is generally only the unbound drug which is biologically active. Therefore, in the case of a highly bound drug, the biological activity resides in only a small proportion of the total plasma level, and a relatively small increase in the unbound fraction may produce a marked increase in therapeutic or toxic activity. Such an increase may result from:

1 a change in concentration of plasma proteins, particularly albumin (in hypoproteinaemic states a higher level of unbound drug occurs in the plasma unless the oral dose is lowered)
2 displacement of bound drug from binding sites on proteins by other drugs

Metabolism

Most drugs are metabolised to some extent in the liver, although, in addition, some are destroyed in the gut wall, plasma and other tissues. Liver metabolism occurs particularly with lipid soluble drugs, which may be taken up so avidly by the liver that a total extraction occurs from the blood during its first passage through the portal circulation after absorption.

The best known example of this 'first pass' phenomenon is propranolol in which between 20 and 40 mg of an oral dose is removed by the liver. Until this hepatic extraction is saturated, little, if any, parent drug is able to reach the systemic circulation. Other drugs with important first-pass effects include morphine and lignocaine.

The object of drug metabolising activity is to produce derivatives of increasing polarity which are less lipid soluble and so more readily excreted by the kidney. Drugs possessing a hydroxyl, carboxyl or amino group are usually conjugated to form a glucuronide, an ethereal sulphate, or a glycine or acetyl derivative. Drugs lacking one of these groups are usually oxidised, dealkylated, deaminated or hydroxylated, and subsequent conjugation often occurs. It is important to remember that a metabolite of a drug may be pharmacologically and therefore therapeutically active, and that its profile of activity may differ from that of the parent drug. This is demonstrated in the case of the tertiary amines amitriptyline and imipramine which are demethylated to the secondary amines nortriptyline and desipramine respectively, both of which are antidepressant drugs, but differ in their pharmacological properties from the parent compounds.

Differences in rates of drug metabolism account for most of the differences in steady-state blood level already referred to. For example, steady-state levels of some MARI antidepressant drugs vary up to 20 or 30 fold on a fixed daily dose, most of this variability being due to differences in rates of hydroxylation, while interpatient differences in protein binding and tissue distribution are two-fold or less.

Acetylation depends on the activity of the enzyme N-acetyl transferase, the concentration of which is genetically determined. The population can be divided into fast and slow acetylators, and this has been shown to influence the therapeutic and toxic effects of a variety of drugs including isoniazid and procainamide. It has been shown that the monoamine oxidase inhibitor phenelzine undergoes acetylation and that clinical response to this drug may depend upon the acetylator status of the patient.

Excretion

Most drugs, or their metabolites, are excreted in the urine, and the same principles apply to passive diffusion through the renal tubule as were discussed earlier with regard to drug absorption. The ionised species of a drug is less lipid soluble and so does not readily diffuse back from the glomerular filtrate through the renal tubular wall into the circulation. Therefore, changes in tubular pH can influence the rate of elimination of weakly acidic or basic drugs and their metabolites. Normally the urine is slightly acid and favours the excretion of weakly basic drugs such as amphetamine, pethidine and tricyclic antidepressants. The reverse applies for weakly acidic drugs, and this is the reason why an alkaline diuresis is used to accelerate the elimination of aspirin and some barbiturates (see chapter 15).

Because the kidney is the main organ of excretion for many drugs, care must be exercised in prescribing drugs for patients with impaired renal function.

Some drugs are excreted mainly in the bile, and may then be reabsorbed from the small bowel to produce an 'entero-hepatic' circulation. Drugs and their metabolites, particularly glucuronide conjugates, are liable to biliary excretion if they are polar and if their molecular weights exceed 400.

Blood levels

Following the absorption of a drug from the gut or from a site of parenteral administration, and its distribution to the tissues, its

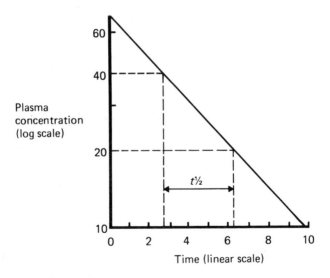

Figure 5 *Hypothetical plot of plasma concentration decline with time*

concentration in the plasma or serum falls along an exponential time course. A semi-logarithmic plot of concentration versus time produces a straight line relationship from which can be obtained the half-life (t½) of the drug, that is, the time taken for the concentration to fall to half of its original level (Figure 5). The half-life, when absorption and distribution is complete, is determined by those processes of metabolism and excretion already described.

The concept of half-life is a valuable one in deciding the frequency of drug dosage. Levodopa, for example, has a short half-life and requires at least four divided doses daily to produce a steady plasma level and therapeutic action. On the other hand, amitriptyline has a half-life of 30–40 hours, and only requires a once-daily administration. The development of a special 'sustained-release' form of this drug for once-nightly administration was, therefore, quite unnecessary. Drugs with a long half-life may be cumulative with repeated and frequent dosage, and patients receiving them should be examined carefully and regularly for signs of overdosage.

The foregoing considerations with respect to blood levels of a drug and its elimination half-life are only of clinical importance when there is a close and temporal relationship between plasma concentration and pharmacological or therapeutic effect. In the case of some centrally acting drugs this clearly applies, for example with lithium. With many others there appears to be a relationship, but it is not so clear-cut, for example with phenothiazine neuroleptics and antidepressant drugs of the monoamine reuptake inhibitor type (MARI). This may be because being very lipid soluble, they reach high concentrations in different parts of the brain, which do not necessarily correlate closely with plasma levels in concentration or time. Finally, there are other drugs whose mechanism of action renders it unlikely that such a close relationship could be found, for example, the monoamine oxidase inhibitors.

Bioavailability

The bioavailability of a drug is the fraction of the administered dose which reaches the systemic circulation without being metabolised. It may be less than unity, either if the drug is not completely absorbed from the gastrointestinal tract because of poor

47

solubility of the drug or an unsatisfactory formulation (see page 42), or if the drug is metabolised in the gut wall (e.g. isoprenaline), the liver (e.g. propranolol, morphine) or the lung (e.g. noradrenaline).

Bioavailability can be calculated by dividing the area under the plasma drug concentration/time curve after oral administration by the area under the curve after intravenous administration of the same dose of drug.

Other factors

Several other factors are recognised which influence drug action, either by effects on the pharmacokinetic variables already mentioned, or by effects on tissue response.

Age has a marked influence on metabolism and excretion particularly at the extremes of life in infancy and old age. Old age brings a reduction in liver metabolising activity and in renal excreting ability. It is also associated with changes in distribution of body tissues, for example, the proportion of body fat. Changes in the cerebral circulation associated with increasing age may also contribute to differences in response to centrally acting drugs seen in elderly patients.

Sex differences almost certainly influence drug activity. Female patients show considerable differences in pressor response to sympathomimetic amines at different times of the menstrual cycle, and this may also apply to central monoamine receptors. Sex differences have been observed in the central stimulation produced by anorectic drugs, which may be due to pharmacokinetic factors as well as to differences in receptor activity.

Drug interactions involving psychotropic drugs

Patients receiving drug treatment for a psychiatric condition are usually receiving more than one drug at the same time, and these may interact in a variety of ways for the patients; either for good or for harm. The following is a summary of some of the mechanisms by which such interactions may take place.

1 Absorption

Drugs which influence the rate of gastric emptying may modify the rate of absorption of other drugs. Anticholinergic activity, in particular, slows the rate of gastric emptying, and this property is shared by several groups of psychotropic drugs including the MARI antidepressant drugs, the phenothiazines, and the anticholinergic antiparkinsonian drugs. Their effect is to delay passage of the drugs into the small bowel, and thus, most commonly, to delay their systemic absorption.

Gut wall and liver monoamine oxidase normally destroys monoamines such as tyramine which is present in food (e.g. in cheese and other foods subject to microbial action) as well as sympathomimetic substances such as phenylephrine which are substrates for the enzyme and are found in proprietary and other medicines used as nasal decongestants and in coryza. Treatment with monoamine oxidase inhibitors reduces the activity of this enzyme and so permits the systemic absorption of such monoamines, with the risk of a hypertensive reaction.

2 Hepatic enzyme induction

The magnitude and duration of action of many drugs, as well as endogenously produced substances, are dependent on their rate of biotransformation by the drug-metabolising enzymes of the liver. The activity of these enzymes may be increased, or induced by treatment with a large number of commonly used substances including insecticides and pesticides, and also by drugs, chiefly the barbiturates, glutethimide, methaqualone, phenytoin and rifampicin. The steady-state plasma concentration of some MARI antidepressant drugs can be markedly reduced by addition of a barbiturate hypnotic to the treatment regimen. Benzodiazepines in therapeutic doses do not induce these enzymes. The state of hepatic drug metabolising activity can be assessed indirectly in vivo by measurement of antipyrine elimination half-lives, serum gamma-glutamyl-transpeptidase, and urinary excretion of glucaric acid and 6-β-hydroxycortisol.

3 Hepatic enzyme inhibition

The effect of monoamine oxidase inhibitors in the gut and liver has already been discussed. Clinically important inhibition of drug metabolising enzymes in the liver may occur with phenothiazines and butyrophenones which may result in reduced metabolism of MARI antidepressants, leading to higher plasma levels and enhanced effects.

4 Blockade of neuronal uptake

The active reuptake of noradrenaline into the neurone is an important mechanism in its termination of action. Blockade of the reuptake process potentiates the pressor action of noradrenaline and adrenaline, and of other drugs that depend on the same uptake process, such as phenylephrine. This may be important in administration of local anaesthetic preparations containing one of these amines as a vasoconstrictor. Among the groups of drugs which may block neuronal uptake are the MARI antidepressants such as amitriptyline and imipramine, and their metabolites nortriptyline and desipramine. Some indirectly acting sympathomimetic amines, such as tyramine, and some adrenergic neurone blocking drugs such as guanethidine, bethanidine and debrisoquine, depend for their pharmacological and therapeutic effects on being taken up into the neurone through the same active uptake process as noradrenaline. Their action may, therefore, be prevented or reversed by treatment with MARI antidepressant drugs. Phenothiazines also possess uptake-blocking properties and may have similar effects on these antihypertensive drugs.

5 Transmitter depletion

The effects of drugs which depend for their action on release of certain transmitter substances may be reduced by administration of other drugs which produce neurotransmitter depletion. For example, pressor responses to tyramine are reduced in reserpinised patients.

6 Functional summation of effects

Drugs which produce a similar pharmacological effect by different mechanisms may have a synergistic interaction; for example, the mutual enhancement in the central nervous system of the depressant activity of hypnotics, sedatives, tranquillisers, alcohol, narcotic analgesics and anaesthetics.

There may also be summation of the same pharmacological effect of several drugs given for different purposes. For example, phenothiazine neuroleptics, many MARI antidepressants, and antiparkinsonian drugs such as orphenadrine and benzhoxol all possess anticholinergic properties which may summate if a member of each group is given together for acceptable psychiatric and neurological indications, to produce a central anticholinergic crisis.

This crisis with its psychological concomitants is sometimes mistaken for worsening of the psychiatric condition for which the psychotropic drugs are being administered; if this happens then higher doses may be prescribed, with potentially disastrous results.

Table 3   *Clinically important interactions involving psychotropic drugs*

Primary drug A	May interact with B	Potential results
Monoamine reuptake inhibitor antidepressant (MARI)	Bethanidine Debrisoquine Guanethidine Clonidine	Reduction of antihypertensive action of B
	Monoamine oxidase inhibitors	Central nervous excitation, hyperyrexia, coma
	Anticholinergics Antihistamines Antiparkinsonian drugs	Excessive central and peripheral atropine-like effects
	Noradrenaline Adrenaline Phenylephrine	Potentiation of pressor action of B
	Any orally administered drug	Change in absorption of B
	Phenothiazines and butyrophenones	Potentiation of hypotensive effect of B

Table 3   *contd.*

Primary drug A	May interact with B	Potential results
Monoamine oxidase inhibitors (MAOI)	Indirectly acting sympathomimetics Fenfluramine Levodopa Foods containing tyramine	Acute adrenergic hypertensive crisis
	MARI antidepressants	Central nervous excitation, hyperpyrexia, coma
	Pethidine	Central nervous excitation, coma
Benzodiazepines	Alcohol Other CNS depressants	Increase CNS depression
Barbiturates	Coumarin anticoagulants	Reduced activity of B
	Corticosteroids	Reduced effect of B in asthma
	Oral contraceptives	Contraceptive failure
	Other CNS depressants	Increase CNS depression
	MARI antidepressants	Reduced plasma levels and ? effect
Beta-adrenoceptor blocking drugs	Antihypertensive drugs	Increased hypotensive action
	Insulin	Increased hypoglycaemic action of B
	Sulphonylureas	
	Skeletal muscle relaxants (depolarising)	Increased activity of B

Table 3   *contd.*

Primary drug *A*	*May interact with* *B*	*Potential results*
Hypnotics	Alcohol Narcotic analgesics Antihistamines MARI antidepressants Phenothiazines Butyrophenones	Increased CNS depression
Phenothiazines and butyrophenones	Alcohol Narcotic analgesics Other CNS depressants	Increased CNS depression
	Anticholinergics	Impaired oral absorption of A
	MARI antidepressants	Enhancement of peripheral and central anticholinergic effects
		? enhanced effect of B through hepatic enzyme inhibition
	Bethanidine Debrisoquine Guanethidine	Reduction of antihypertensive action of B
Lithium	Diuretics	Lithium retention and toxicity
	Sodium chloride	With reduced sodium intake, lithium retention. With increased sodium intake, greater lithium excretion

Suggestions for further reading

Pharmacokinetics

CURRY, S. H., *Drug Disposition and Pharmacokinetics*, 2nd edn, Blackwell, Oxford, 1977.

DAVIES, D. S., and PRICHARD, B. N. C., *Biological Effect of Drugs in Relation to their Plasma Concentration*, Macmillan, London, 1973.

GIBALDI, M., *Biopharmaceutics and Clinical Pharmacokinetics*, Lea and Febiger, 1984.

JOHNSTONE, E., and MARSH, W., 'Acetylator status and response to phenelzine in depressed patients', *Lancet*, vol. 1, 1973, p. 567.

SCHANKER, L. S., 'Physiological transport of drugs', in *Advances in Drug Research*, ed. N. J. Harper and A. B. Simmonds, Academic Press, London, 1965, vol. 1, p. 71.

SMITH, S. E., and RAWLINS, M. D., *Variability in Human Drug Response*, Butterworths, London, 1973.

TURNER, P., and RICHENS, A., *Clinical Pharmacology*, 5th edn, Churchill Livingstone, Edinburgh, 1986.

VESSEL, E. S., 'Pharmacogenetics', *Biochemical Pharmacology*, vol. 24, 1975, p. 445.

WAGNER, J. G., *Fundamentals of Clinical Pharmacokinetics*, Drug Intelligence Publications, Hamilton, Illinois, 1975.

Drug interactions

BEELEY, L., *Safer Prescribing*, 4th edn, Blackwell, Oxford, 1987.

DAVIES, D. M., *Textbook of Adverse Drug Reactions*, 2nd edn, Oxford University Press, 1981.

TURNER, P., and RICHENS, A., *Clinical Pharmacology*, 5th edn, Churchill Livingstone, Edinburgh, 1986.

Methods of studying behavioural effects of drugs   4

In most other areas of clinical pharmacology the therapeutic effects
of a new drug may be predicted with some confidence on the basis
of animal experiments alone. However, in psychopharmacology it
is difficult to predict behavioural effects in man from findings
obtained in animals. This is because:

1 there are few, if any, satisfactory animal models of abnormal
  human mental states such as schizophrenia, depression, mania
  or anxiety;
2 it is often impossible to be certain whether objective changes in
  animal behaviour after administration of a drug are due to
  sensory or motor effects, or both, or to changes in coordination,
  or even to hallucinatory effects.

In fact, it may not be possible to detect any therapeutic drug
effect at all until the compound is given to patients suffering with a
particular condition. For example, levodopa has few, if any, central
effects in normal subjects but can readily be seen to affect motor
activity in patients with Parkinson's disease. Similarly, the clinical
activity of the antidepressant group of drugs can only be detected
in patients with established depressive illness. Although valuable
clues may come from various animal tests, these tests often appear
to bear little relation to clinical conditions in man.

In this chapter, tests will be briefly described which may be used
to detect and evaluate central actions of drugs in animals and man,
particularly those drugs to which reference will be made in later
sections of the book.

Animal tests

There are a very large number of animal tests used to screen the
effects of drugs on the central nervous system, and to study their

mechanism of action. They can be classified in three main groups:

1 Pharmacological and biochemical
2 Behavioural
3 Electroneurophysiological

1 *Pharmacological and biochemical tests*

These include biochemical and histochemical studies of animal brain tissue to demonstrate localisation of possible transmitter substances and the influence of drugs upon them, as well as test procedures involving isotopically labelled drugs, such as auto-radiography (to show the distribution of a drug within various organs) and tracer studies (to determine the metabolic pathway of a drug).

A commonly used test for screening potential antidepressant compounds makes use of reserpine-induced hypothermia. Administration of reserpine to an animal reduces its body temperature, probably by monoamine depletion. MAO inhibitors and dibenza-zepine derivatives, known to have antidepressant activity in man, reverse this hypothermic effect of reserpine. On the other hand, some other types of antidepressant drugs such as mianserin do not possess this property.

2 *Behavioural tests*

There are a large number of tests in which the effects of drugs on animal behaviour may be observed. These can range from simple observation of turning behaviour in a rat in which the substantia nigra has been destroyed, to the detailed analysis of social interaction in pairs of laboratory animals. The first type of test is designed to explore neurochemical mechanisms underlying drug actions; in the example given it is to examine the role of dopaminergic systems in the actions of certain drugs such as levodopa and haloperidol on motor behaviour. The second type of test is designed to model as far as possible the clinical effects of psychotropic drugs.

It has been proposed that any animal model of a psychiatric disorder should fulfil the following criteria:

1 The situations which induce the behaviour observed in the animal model should resemble in general terms the situations which induce the clinical state in man.
2 The behaviour of the animal should show features analogous to those in the clinical condition being modelled.
3 The neurobiological mechanisms should be similar in both the animal model and the clinical state.
4 The change in behaviour observed in the animal model should be reversed by treatments known to be effective in ameliorating the clinical condition under consideration.

Although a number of cogent criticisms have been levelled against these criteria, and in fact against animal models in general, such models do allow investigation of the neural mechanisms believed to be involved in the pathogenesis of certain psychiatric disorders. Furthermore, information obtained from studies of the effects of drugs on animal behaviour might suggest novel hypotheses and treatments for clinical conditions.

Thus far, anxiety-related conditions are those for which the most relevant animal models have been developed, although 'learned helplessness' in dogs is thought by some to reflect depressive states. For the study of anxiety and antianxiety drugs the most appropriate model is the social interaction test. In this test pairs of male rats are placed in familiar conditions in low illuminosity (low stress) where they show high levels of social interaction, and in unfamiliar conditions in high illuminosity (high stress) where they show low levels of social interaction. Drugs such as chlordiazepoxide, which is an effective antianxiety drug in man, increase the amount of social interaction seen in the high stress situation to the levels observed in the low stress situations; thus they appear to exert an antianxiety effect, which, in this test, can be clearly distinguished from any non-specific sedative effect they may have.

3 *Electroneurophysiological tests*

Neuronal activity within the brain and spinal cord is accompanied by changes in electrical potential across the cell membrane. The summation of these changes in large numbers of neurones may be recorded by superficial electrodes placed on the scalp, as in electroencephalography, a technique widely used in human studies. In animals it is possible to implant electrodes in specific areas of the brain, or even localise them to individual cells, and so record electrical events more discretely.

A sophisticated modification of this principle involves introducing a minute amount of pharmacologically active substance in the vicinity of a neurone through a micropipette controlled by micromanipulators, and recording the potential changes produced with adjacent microelectrodes. Multichannel micropipettes have been developed by drawing out a number of glass tubes fixed together. The multichannel micropipette made in this way has closely adjacent openings at the common tip, the central channel of which may be used as a recording electrode, while the secondary pipettes can be used for the introduction of substances whose actions are to be tested. For recording extracellular potentials in the brain it is preferable to use electrodes with a tip diameter of 6 μ or less.

As well as recording electrical changes in the brain and spinal cord, implanted electrodes may be used to stimulate discrete areas and study the effects of such stimulation on the animal's behaviour and physiology. The influence of drugs on such responses to electrical stimulation may then be investigated.

Tests in man

It is essential to test the effects of centrally acting drugs on psychomotor function in human subjects in order to know how such drugs are likely to effect complex behaviours such as those required to drive a motor car in traffic or to handle potentially dangerous industrial machinery. A number of testing procedures of different levels of complexity have been designed for this purpose using one of two basic approaches. One approach is to build up a profile of a given drug's effects in a variety of laboratory tests, to assess specific skills. The other is to examine the effect of drugs on complex behaviours using simulators or low-speed car handling tasks. Even such complicated procedures may not detect subtle effects on judgment and decision making, impairment of which are a much more frequent cause of accidents than lack of motor skills. When carrying out such testing procedures it is essential to take account of the pharmacokinetics of the drug in question (see chapter 3) and to make repeated measures of the effects of a range of doses over time.

Sensory tests

1 *Critical flicker fusion* A test of visual function which is mediated by the central nervous system, and is most useful in the monitoring of drug effects on the brain, is the critical flicker frequency (CFF). This may be defined as the fastest rate at which a flashing source of light appears to be flickering as opposed to being steady. It has a number of determinants including the luminance, wave-length, wave-form and light–dark ratio of the stimulating light; the area, portion and light-adapted state of the retina illuminated; the duration of exposure, and the size of the pupil. Age and constitutional factors may also influence the threshold and recently the importance of intersensory effects has been recognised.

By rigorously controlling these many variables in the experimental situation it has been possible to use the test for assessing the effects of central depressant and stimulant drugs. Alcohol produces a marked depression of CFF which is proportional to the alcohol concentration in blood and urine. Barbiturate drugs depress CFF and dose response effects may be obtained starting with doses as low as 50 mg amylobarbitone. Antianxiety drugs, such as meprobamate, chlordiazepoxide and diazepam, as well as phenothiazine drugs, lower CFF in doses which are too small to produce any subjective awareness of central depression. Indeed, CFF is one of the most sensitive measures currently available for detecting the effects of centrally acting drugs in healthy human subjects.

Central stimulant drugs such as amphetamine and phenmetrazine increase CFF, as do hallucinogenic stimulant compounds such as psylocybin. Combinations of barbiturates and amphetamines in appropriate proportions may show mutual antagonism of effects on CFF. Thus, a mixture of dexamphetamine and amylobarbitone in the proportions found in Drinamyl produces no change in CFF when compared with placebo, although dexamphetamine alone produces a rise and amylobarbitone a fall in threshold. Measurement of CFF over a period of time allows a study of the duration of action of drugs and the influence of physiological variables on it. For example, the rate of excretion of amphetamine is markedly dependent on urinary pH, a low pH resulting in rapid elimination of the drug and an alkaline urine delaying its excretion. A comparison of the duration of action of amphetamine on CFF under conditions of urinary acidity and alkalinity showed that the magnitude and duration of elevation of CFF was significantly greater under alkaline than under acid conditions.

Drugs may also affect the peripheral components of vision such as extraocular motor balance, pupil and lens function and rod and cone activity involved in colour vision.

2 *Hearing* Just as the critical flicker frequency is a measure of a subject's ability to distinguish an intermittent light source, so the auditory flutter-fusion threshold (AFFT) is a measure of central auditory function. An interrupted random noise signal is used, and although the threshold varies greatly from subject to subject, it is very constant for any one person if measured, like the CFF, under strictly controlled conditions. Amylobarbitone 100 mg, diazepam 10 mg and chlorpromazine 25 mg and 50 mg significantly depress the AFFT, while amphetamine 10 mg raises it.

Auditory vigilance tasks have been developed which can be made extremely sensitive to drug effects. In one such test subjects listen to 1 kHz tones of 82 dB against a background white noise of 76 dB. The duration of the tone is usually 0.5 sec but shorter tones of 0.4 sec are randomly presented as critical stimuli to be recognised by pressing a button.

Tests of coordination and motor function

It is difficult to draw fine distinctions between sensory, motor and coordination tests in man, for even the sensory tests already described require a response from the subject which involves some coordination and motor activity. Nevertheless, in the tests previously described, the emphasis was mainly on sensory activity, whereas in the tests described in this section, attention is focused primarily on motor skills and on coordination of motor with sensory activity. It may not be easy to distinguish, however, between effects of drugs on local neuromuscular and spinal activity, and effects on the brain. Furthermore, the potential effects of motivation and of learning must be taken into account; it is usually advisable when testing drugs in volunteer subjects to train them until the response measure has reached a limiting value before examining the effects of the drug on performance.

1 *Reaction time* The simple reaction time is the time taken for a subject to record a response to a given stimulus. In an alert subject this time may be very short, and electronic timing devices may be required to give a sufficiently accurate measurement. Even before the introduction of such equipment, however, it was possible to obtain results which showed effects of central depressant drugs. A century ago Lauder Brunton used a system of pendulums and levers to demonstrate the effects of alcohol and other drugs on central function. The simple reaction time is relatively insensitive to drug effects and it is now customary to use a method to determine *choice reaction time* when evaluating the effects of a centrally acting drug on psychomotor function. Here the subject is presented with a number of stimuli, usually four or five, and can make a number of possible responses usually by pressing different keys. As generally administered, the subject is instructed to respond to only one of the stimuli by pressing one specific key. This test is quite sensitive to centrally acting drugs.

2 *Disc dotting* In this test of coordination, in which the McDougal–Schuster machine is most commonly used, a subject cancels, with a pencil, an irregular spiral of dots within circles as it rotates slowly on a turntable. Vision is restricted by covering the spiral with a lid in which there is only a small radial aperture. The cancellations begin at the origin of the spiral at the centre of the turntable and continue until the subject misses two consecutive target circles; the score comprises the number of 'dots' in the track up to the point where it has been broken.

A modification of this method consists of a rotating metal drum covered with an insulating layer in which holes have been cut in an irregular spiral course. The subject uses a steering-wheel to follow the course of holes with a lever and thus establishes electrical contact with them; the score is recorded on a digital counter. Drugs such as promethazine when given in single doses, have been shown to reduce performance significantly.

3 *Number cancellation* This relatively simple paper and pencil test is useful for examining the effects of drugs on the perceptional process of sensory information. In this type of test a random series of digits is presented in which the particular digit to be cancelled appears a predetermined number of times, and the number of the

61

digits cancelled in a set time (usually ninety seconds) is counted. This test is quite sensitive to low doses of sedative drugs.

4 *Digit symbol substitution* This test, which forms part of the Wechsler Adult Intelligence Test battery, can be regarded as another test of perceptual processing, but one which makes rather more demands on central integrative mechanisms; it also contains a motor component. In this test a subject is asked to substitute given symbols for individual numbers according to a predetermined code; alternatively numbers can be substituted for symbols. One advantage of this test is that a large number of alternative forms are possible, reducing the possibility of learning effects markedly influencing the result.

5 *Tapping speed* This is a test of both coordination and motor ability, in which the subject taps on a morse key as rapidly as possible for a given period of time; a counter registers the number of contacts made.

6 *Hand steadiness* There are a variety of test situations designed to measure hand steadiness. Most require the subject to hold a metal rod or ring in close proximity to another metal object, such as a plate or wire, or to move one along the other, without allowing the two to touch. Contact of the metal objects completes an electrical circuit which can activate a bell, buzzer or light. The apparatus may be designed to give the subject a harmless but unpleasant shock when this happens.

7 *Pursuit rotor* In this test a point light source moves rapidly on a screen and the subject attempts to follow it with a rod at the end of which is a photoelectric cell. This records the amount of time for which the subject is able to keep the rod in contact with the light source and hence the accuracy of this movement.

8 *Reverse mirror drawing* This is a measure, not only of a subject's coordination, but also his sense of lateralisation. He sees the image of a design, such as a star, in a mirror in front of him, but the design itself is hidden by a screen. He is required to follow the outline of the design with a pencil held below the screen, controlling it from the mirror image. The time taken to complete the test, and the number of errors made, are recorded.

9 *Simulators* Simulators have been designed to replicate as closely as possible the sensory experience of being in a car or aeroplane and to make demands on the operator of a similar nature to those he or she would experience when driving or flying. Centrally acting drugs, particularly benzodiazepines have been found to affect performance in such situations.

10 *Low-speed car handling* Despite their apparent similarity to the real situation, car simulators can only at best be an approximation to driving a car, especially driving a car in traffic. To overcome this limitation several investigators have studied the effects of drugs on car handling in a gymkhana-like situation where the operator is instructed to drive into and reverse out of a 'garage', to park parallel to the kerb, and to negotiate a slalom course of upright poles. Even relatively small doses of certain benzodiazepines have been shown to impair car-handling ability in these tests.

Psychological rating scales

Psychotropic drugs are usually prescribed for the relief of emotional distress or the amelioration of a disturbed mental state; two conditions which are very difficult to measure directly. To determine the relative efficacy of such drugs in these clinical situations we have to rely on a variety of rating scales, and other psychometric tests, a number of which are available. They fall into four broad categories:

1 Tests of intelligence and other cognitive functions
2 Scales designed to quantify overt behaviour
3 Ratings based on a standardised clinical interview
4 Self-rating scales completed by the patient himself

1 *Intelligence tests and other tests of cognitive function* These are perhaps the most familiar of all psychological measuring devices having been in use for over fifty years. Essentially, they attempt to quantify the ability of the subject to solve standardised problems and to learn new information. They are particularly useful in cases of suspected organic disease of the brain, and the most commonly used are the Wechsler Adult Intelligence Scale (WAIS), the progressive matrices, and the Mill Hill Vocabulary Test.

63

2 *Overt behaviour scales* These scales are among the earliest introduced for specifically psychiatric purposes. Among the first was the Phipps Psychiatric Clinic Behaviour Chart introduced in 1915 for nurses to use in making a daily numerical assessment of a variety of behaviours exhibited by their patients on the ward. A more recent example of this type of scale is in the Nurses' Observation For Inpatient Evaluation (NOSIE).

The disadvantages of such measures are: first, they can be used only on hospital in-patients, and then only in a ward where the numbers and training of the nursing staff are adequate; and second, they afford very little information on subjective phenomena such as emotions, perceptions and beliefs.

3 *Clinical rating scales* These are basically designed to provide a quantitative estimate of the findings obtained during a clinical interview. There are two types, each having a somewhat different aim:

(i) Scales designed to provide information over a wide range of possible symptoms; they are useful as an aid to diagnosis.
(ii) Scales which are primarily intended for estimating changes in individual symptoms occurring in specific psychiatric disorders.

While the second group of scales is only valid after a diagnosis has been made, it does allow more critical evaluation of drug changes within the particular given diagnostic grouping under study.

The complexity of rating scales of the first type ranges from the sixteen-item *Brief Psychiatric Rating Scale* to the *Present Psychiatric State Examination* covering over 400 items.

For any rating scale to be clinically useful it must have both validity and reliability.

(i) Validity refers to its potential to measure what it is intended to measure. In the case of rating scales for use in the assessment of drug treatments this would refer to the question of a change in score reflecting a change in the underlying severity of the condition under investigation. In practice, since there is no objective measure against which the scale can be unequivocally validated, validation becomes a matter of comparing the change observed in two different measures during the same period (concurrent validity), or of comparing the scores in a group of patients expressing clinical symptoms to those observed in a group of normal volunteers or patients who have become symptom free (construct validity).

(ii) Reliability is a measure of the stability of a rating scale. This can reflect the closeness of score obtained by two independent raters on the same occasion (inter-rater reliability), or the consistency of score obtained by the same rater on different occasions (test–retest reliability). However, when the clinical condition changes as a result of treatment, examination of test–retest reliability is not possible as any change in the score from one occasion to another may reflect a true change in clinical status rather than any unreliability of the test in question.

Finally, it should be stressed that there is no intrinsic numerical value in the scores obtained by any of these scales; they merely enable a clinical impression or a subjective feeling state to be quantified. They do not actually measure anything directly.

4 *Self-rating scales* With this type of scale, which does not require the presence of either a doctor, a psychologist or a nurse, the patient himself completes it by answering a series of multiple-choice questions. Here is a sample question from a self-rating scale used in the assessment of depression, the *Beck Depression Scale* (only one of the following statements must be marked as reflecting the patient's feelings):

0 I do not feel sad.
1 I feel blue and sad.
2a I am blue and sad all the time and I can't snap out of it.
2b I am so sad or unhappy that it is very painful.
3 I am so sad or unhappy that I can't stand it.

While such scales are obviously open to evasion or exaggeration by patients, in practice they are extremely useful and are economical of professional time.

The major difficulty encountered by patients completing such scales is the inability to decide upon one particular answer or category. (These scales are often referred to as *category scales*.) This is especially true of the Yes/No-type scales such as the *Eysenck Personality Inventory* (EPI), a very widely used measure intended to obtain an assessment of personality in terms of neuroticism, extraversion and introversion.

An innovation which avoids this difficulty is the *Visual Analogue*

Scale consisting of a straight line, usually 100 mm long, one end labelled, for example, 'not at all anxious' and the other 'extremely anxious'. The labels can vary according to the condition or sensation being evaluated. Patients are asked to mark the line at the point which most appropriately reflects their state at the time. While there is considerable variation in the way different people use such a scale, it allows a very sensitive assessment of change occurring within a given person, and is particularly useful in monitoring drug effects.

Choice of rating scale

1 *For screening and diagnosis* The choice of rating scale for any given project depends partly on the purpose for which it is to be used, and partly on the clinical condition to be studied. It is in most cases a compromise between exhaustiveness and exhaustion. If a great deal of information is required about a relatively small number of patients, and there are sufficient trained personnel to administer the scale, then the *Present State Examination* is without doubt the most comprehensive available instrument. However, most clinical studies of psychotropic drugs require relatively large numbers of patients and take place in clinics and hospitals where staff time is at a premium. Therefore for out-patient and general practice investigations, self-rating scales such as the *General Health Questionnaire* are more useful.

2 *For assessment of severity* A number of rating scales have been designed to assess the severity of a particular syndrome at repeated points in time. Such scales have a wide application in psychopharmacology, allowing the efficacy of various drug treatments to be quantified and compared.

For most syndromes there are available both self-rating scales and clinician rating scales. In those conditions where the symptoms are causing the patient concern and distress, self-rating scales are more appropriate; these would include anxiety states, phobias and minor depressive episodes. In more serious psychiatric disturbance, such as mania, schizophrenia or severe depressive illness, clinician rating scales are preferable, as patients suffering from these conditions are frequently unable, by reason of their illness, to complete self-rating scales. Some of the more widely employed and useful rating scales are listed in Table 4.

Table 4   *Clinical rating scales*

	Self-administered	*Observer rated*
Screening and diagnosis	General Health Questionnaire	Present State Examination
	Hopkins Symptom Checklist	Clinical Interview Schedule
		Geriatric Mental State Schedule
Depression	Beck Depression Inventory	Hamilton Depression Rating Scale
	Wakefield Self-assessment Depression Inventory	Montgomery-Asberg Depression Rating Scale
	Zung Self-rating Depression Scale	
Mania		Bech-Rafaelson Mania Scale
		Petterson Mania Rating Scale
		Young Mania Scale
Schizophrenia		Brief Psychiatric Rating Scale
		Krawiecka Scale
		Montgomery Schizophrenia Scale
Anxiety	Taylor Manifest Anxiety Scale	Hamilton Anxiety Rating Scale
	Morbid Anxiety Inventory	
Dementia		Information – Memory – Concentration Test

Psychophysiological tests

Many psychiatric disorders are accompanied by physical manifestations. Centrally acting drugs may affect these manifestations, or may themselves have direct effects on various physiological activities. Only a brief review of some of the test procedures used in this field of psychophysiological measurement will be attempted here.

1 *Heart rate and blood pressure* Heart rate and blood pressure may be abnormal in psychotic conditions, such as depression, mania and anxiety. Centrally acting drugs may also produce changes in these parameters, either through their central effect or through other peripheral actions which they possess.

In some circumstances it may be sufficient to record pulse rate by simply counting the radial pulse for a minute, and to measure blood pressure by the standard sphygmomanometer technique, after the subject has rested for at least five minutes. However, for a more accurate assessment of drugs on central and peripheral autonomic function, it is preferable to use electrical recording devices. While a standard electrocardiogram (ECG) will provide sufficient data to record heart rate, it does not provide the information in a useful way. By employing electronic circuits to perform the operations involved in heart beat recognition, counting and timing, by using a cardiotachometer, the need to count individual ECG complexes is avoided. Introduction of newer techniques based on the measurement of systolic time intervals using a high speed surface ECG provide even more sensitive measures. In particular such techniques allow earlier detection of any potential cardiotoxic effects a particular psychotropic drug may have.

Automated recording of systolic and diastolic levels of blood pressure is more difficult, and in fact, there are few, if any, accurate methods which do not depend on arterial catheterisation, although systolic blood pressure alone may be recorded with rather simpler techniques. A commonly used method involves occlusion of the blood supply to a finger, using a small cuff. The point of occlusion is then determined by testing for a pulse distal to the cuff by means of: (i) a second cuff connected to a sensitive volume-displacement transducer, (ii) a small finger plethysmograph, (iii) a small crystal transducer strapped to the finger tip, (iv) by observing changes in optical density of the finger tip photoelectrically. Refinements of these methods permit continuous and automatic recording of systolic pressure.

The *Tyramine Pressor Response Test* provides a sensitive guide to the effect psychotropic drugs have on blood pressure when interacting with tyramine containing foodstuffs; this latter aspect assumes particular importance with monoamine oxidase inhibitors (see chapter 7). The test consists of the administration of incremental doses of tyramine until the systolic blood pressure rises to 30 mm Hg above baseline. From the dose response curve obtained the dose of tyramine required to raise the systolic blood pressure by 30 mm Hg after treatment with the drug in question, is compared to the dose of tyramine required to raise blood pressure to the same degree after placebo.

2 *Skin conductance and skin potential* When a small electric current is passed between two points on the surface of the skin the conductance varies with the state of the subject's mental state. Measurements of the skin conductance levels are usually made over the palm; they often show slow and gradual changes as a function of the changing mental state of the individual; in the case of sleeping or drugged subjects the conductance may fall markedly, while the conductance rises rapidly following specific arousing stimuli.

Measurement of skin conductance changes are of considerable value in psychopharmacology, including the so-called psycho-galvanic response (PGR) in which there is a change in conductance occurring as a result of a psychological stimulus. The technique is not simple, however, for the voltage and conductance involved is small, and requires sophisticated electronic recording apparatus and intimate electrode–skin contact to obtain accurate measurement. In addition, the stimuli used must be carefully controlled in order to keep arousal levels as constant as possible. Furthermore, it should be remembered that changes in skin conductance can occur with drugs which influence sweat gland function by a purely peripheral action.

3 *Plethysmography* Plethysmography consists of enclosing an organ in a rigid container called an oncometer and measuring the volume changes of the enclosed part. This permits study of the

nervous and chemical control of blood flow into the organ and changes in that blood flow induced by disease or drugs.

There are many different kinds of plethysmograph, but those used in psychopharmacology usually involve recording pulsatile variations in the volume of a finger or the forearm. Although these measurements of variations in organ volume are not direct estimations of rate of blood flow, under certain strictly controlled conditions, which usually involve sudden occlusion of the venous drainage, the pulse volume is a close index of the rate of blood flow.

Plethysmography is used particularly in studies of anxiety, mania and depression, in which physiological changes in blood flow can be demonstrated, and in the effects of drugs in these conditions.

Penile plethysmography is a variant of the method in which volume changes of the penis during erection can be determined by measuring the changes in a mercury-filled loop placed around the penis. This technique is of particular value when assessing the effect of various treatments on sexual responsiveness, as, for example, in the treatment of sexual deviance by cyproterone.

4 *Electromyography* Tension of a muscle at rest can be a valuable indicator of the mental state of a subject, particularly in conditions of stress and agitation. Although direct measurement of muscle tension in man is difficult, the electrical changes which accompany muscle activity can be recorded; it is also possible to record muscle tremor by suitable modification of the procedure. Electromyograms are usually obtained from surface electrodes placed over appropriate muscle groups but may be complicated by artefacts which make interpretation difficult. An alternative method is to use needle electrodes, but the major difficulty here is that only a very small volume of muscle tissue is sampled by the electrode tip and its precise localisation may not be easy to determine.

5 *Electroencephalography* A detailed discussion of the changes which can occur in the electroencephalogram (EEG) in mental and neurological disease, or in response to drugs, is beyond the scope of this book. Many physiological and metabolic variables influence the EEG and considerable experience is required to recognise changes which are due to extraneous factors. However, the EEG changes produced by certain groups of drugs are so consistent that

their presence in a record can be considered as a strong indication that such drugs have been taken. Stopping drugs, particularly when the subject has become habituated to them, may also affect the EEG in important ways. For example, paroxysmal discharges may be seen in a significant proportion of subjects following barbiturate withdrawal, even in the absence of any previous history of epilepsy.

Because of the large number of variables which may modify the EEG, the following strictly controlled conditions are required for recording:

1 Complete routine EEG assessment, including sleep records, should be made on all supposedly normal subjects before admission to a study
2 All records should be taken by the same recorder
3 The same EEG apparatus should be used throughout
4 Subjects should be investigated at the same time of day and at the same time interval after the previous meal
5 Females should be investigated at the same stage of the menstrual cycle
6 Recording techniques should be standardised
7 Quantitative measurements based on short samples of the EEG should be made at a constant time interval after eye closure or eye opening

It is most convenient to use computerised methods of frequency analysis and summation to demonstrate changes in the EEG. A valuable additional technique measures 'evoked potentials', which are EEG responses evoked by specific stimuli such as visual or auditory signals. Many evoked potentials are of low amplitude and obscured by spontaneous background activity. However, as they are of a constant pattern, frequency analysis and summation procedures allow them to be picked out more clearly. The influence of drugs on these evoked potentials is of considerable interest.

6 *Brain-imaging techniques* In recent years a number of highly sophisticated imaging techniques have been developed for detecting abnormalities and changes in the intact human brain. That which is of the greatest potential interest to the clinical psychopharmacologist is positron emission tomography (PET). PET uses as its basic principle the measurement of emitted positrons from short-lived isotopes such as ^{11}C, ^{18}N, ^{15}O and ^{18}F. Chemical

compounds relevant to CNS function are labelled with these isotopes which are produced in a cyclotron shortly before use. PET is likely to increase significantly our understanding of the neurochemical processes underlying the therapeutic actions of psychotropic drugs in the very near future, and has already been successfully applied to studying the interaction of dopamine receptors blocking drugs with dopamine receptors in normal volunteers and in patients suffering from schizophrenia.

7 *Pupillometry* Changes in pupil size are continuously taking place in association with alterations in mood and response to emotional stimuli. Arousal and fear produce pupillary dilatation while revulsion and disgust produce contraction. Centrally acting drugs, as well as drugs which modify peripheral autonomic activity, may also influence pupil size.

The pupil is supplied by both sympathetic and parasympathetic divisions of the autonomic nervous system and its diameter is readily measurable by photographic and other methods. Its responses to drugs, such as cholinergic and sympathomimetic substances, are consistent in repeated determination within subjects under standard conditions.

There are several methods available for measuring pupil responses. When rapid changes in diameter are being recorded, and when pupillary reactivity to light and dark is also being observed, infra-red pupillography is the most convenient. Infra-red light is reflected from the retina through the pupil, and is then monitored continuously on a recording apparatus, to show pupillary contraction and dilatation.

Where slower responses are being studied, however, this is often unnecessary and simpler photographic methods are equally acceptable; photographs of the eyes are taken and pupil diameter measured from the negatives after suitable magnification.

Among the centrally acting drugs which have been studied in this way, dibenzazepine derivatives such as imipramine produce pupil dilatation due, in part, if not completely, to reduced parasympathetic activity. Phenothiazines, butyrophenones and reserpine contract the pupil to varying extents. Pupillary response to locally instilled sympathomimetic amines may be influenced by centrally acting drugs, and this may provide valuable information on their basic pharmacological actions. For example, oral reserpine treatment reduces or may even abolish the mydriatic action of the indirectly acting amines ephedrine, amphetamine and tyramine while leaving the direct effects of phenylephrine unchanged. On the other hand, treatment with monoamine oxidase inhibitors potentiates the mydriatic actions of the indirectly acting amines.

8 *Feeding behaviour* Feeding behaviour and appetite are affected in many psychiatric conditions and influenced by a number of centrally acting drugs (see chapter 12). Hunger can be reliably assessed with a visual analogue scale (see above). Food intake, on the other hand, while easier to measure directly, presents technical difficulties of application. Many studies on food intake have in fact been limited to the measurement of liquid nutriments such as Metercal (Metrecal). Recently, however, a food dispenser has been developed which allows of the continuous monitoring of the intake of solid foods presented in acceptable standard aliquots.

Clinical trials

In psychiatric disease states, where there are virtually no appropriate animal models, potential therapeutic compounds can only be fully evaluated in patients. In addition, as there are so relatively few parameters in these conditions which can be measured accurately enough to assess the effects of drugs, and as the natural history may be unpredictable, it becomes difficult to relate change in clinical state to the effects of the treatment given.

For all these reasons it is important to design well-controlled clinical trials in order to evaluate the action of centrally acting drugs in psychiatry.

It must be emphasised that a clinical trial is essentially an experiment to investigate the efficacy, safety and acceptability of a given treatment. In common with other clinical experiments, a clinical trial is a compromise between what is desirable theoretically and what is possible practically.

Clinical trials of new drugs are of four main types which have been categorised as Phases I, II, III and IV.

Phase I trials

These are primarily concerned with safety, bioavailability and pharmacokinetics. Such trials are carried out first of all in normal volunteer subjects in a range of age groups, and subsequently in suitable patients.

In this type of trial, which may include the first administration of a new drug to man, a relatively small number of subjects are studied in depth. The drug is first administered in very small doses to normal subjects, with informed consent having been obtained. Test procedures such as those already described in this chapter are carried out before and at intervals after administration of the drug, together with toxicological studies, including haematology, liver and renal function, and electrocardiography. The toxicological tests are done at suitable times to show acute effects and to reveal any delayed hypersensitivity reactions which may occur. Metabolic and biochemical studies provide information on the absorption, excretion and biotransformation of the drug.

Phase II trials

These are studies involving a relatively small number of patients to determine whether the drug has any beneficial effect on the conditions for which it is being given, and if so at what dose. In addition it should be possible by carefully monitoring any unwanted effects to determine a therapeutic index for the drug. That is, the ratio of the efficacy of the drug in question to its tendency to cause undesirable side effects or toxic reactions when administered at what appears to be an effective dose.

Phase III trials

These are what are generally referred to as controlled trials. They are designed to answer the following questions: (i) Has the compound significant therapeutic effects when compared with an identical placebo preparation? (ii) Is the new treatment as good as, or superior to, the best treatment at present available? The answer to the first question will tell whether the drug is therapeutically active when investigator and subject bias have been excluded. Even if it were active, it would have little place in clinical practice if it were shown to be inferior to treatment already available. The controlled clinical trial is an experimental technique by which reliable answers to both these questions can be obtained.

Bias on the part of the investigator or patient is a major source of error in the assessment of psychopharmacological agents. Many

Table 5   *Effect of research design on the outcome of clinical trials*

Research design	Studies reporting less than 70% patients improving no. %	Studies reporting 70% or more improving no. %
No control groups or blind techniques	93 (42)	127 (58)
Control groups but no blind techniques	57 (54)	48 (46)
Control groups and blind techniques	66 (67)	32 (33)

From *Psychopharmacology Bulletin*, March 1969

studies have shown that the greater the degree of control introduced into a trial of a new drug, and the smaller the opportunity for bias, the less enthusiastic are the claims made for it; these findings are illustrated in Table 5.

The most important measures taken to eliminate bias are (1) the double-blind technique, (2) randomisation of treatments and (3) matching of patients.

1   *Double-blind technique*   The purpose of this technique is to ensure that neither investigator nor patient is aware of the treatment which the patient is receiving. For each treatment the new drug, a standard drug and an inactive placebo, are prepared in such a way that they appear identical. This may simply mean making tablets of the same colour, shape and size, but it may also involve flavouring to match the taste, and even introducing other substances to produce unrelated drug effects. For example, if a trial of a new dibenzazepine derivative is to be really double-blind, all the treatments used should produce some impairment of accommodation, dryness of mouth and interference with micturition and bowel function.

An important consideration when preparing a double-blind trial is to ensure that the formulation of the standard drug, which is usually a compound in current use, provides the same 'biological availability' as the generally used preparation. Otherwise, another error might be introduced, loading the result unfairly in favour of, or against, the new drug (see page 47).

2 *Randomisation of treatments* Having disguised the various treatments used in a study, it is important that the order of allocation be randomised.

Trials may be divided broadly into those (i) *within subjects* and those (ii) *between subjects*. In within-subject trials, all the patients receive each of the treatments being tested, and their responses to each treatment are compared to their responses to the other treatments. In between-subject investigations, each patient receives only one of the treatments under trial, and the mean responses of each group of patients receiving a particular treatment are compared to the mean responses of the other groups. Which type of trial is used depends primarily on the nature of the condition being treated. In a chronic condition, such as hypertension or rheumatoid arthritis, a within-patient study is suitable because patients may be expected to return to a similar base-line of disability when treatment is discontinued. However, in conditions which are self-limiting or cyclic in nature, such as the common cold, anxiety states or depression, this assumption cannot be made, and it is not reasonable to compare treatments within the same patient.

Randomisation of treatments is necessary in both within- and between-subjects types of trial. There are two important reasons for this:

(i) It avoids observer bias. If the investigator knows the order of administration of treatment, or that C regularly follows B which follows A, then the trial cannot be considered double-blind, even though the formulations used have been matched for factors such as colour, size and shape. Claims based on trials in which treatments with active drug and placebo were allocated alternately have not been substantiated when trials with true randomisation were undertaken.

(ii) It minimises 'carry-over' effects. The administration of one drug may influence the action of subsequent treatments in a variety of ways and so disguise their true effects. This is particularly important, of course, in within-subject trials. It is overcome by using the 'latin square' type of randomisation. This is best explained by imagining that we have our three preparations, standard, new and placebo. Subjects are arranged in blocks of three, each of whom will have a first, second and third treatment. The latin square is so arranged that each preparation occurs once, and once only, as first, second or third treatment in any three patients, as shown:

$$
\begin{array}{ccc}
A & B & C \\
B & C & A \\
C & A & B
\end{array}
$$

It is evident that in the case of three treatments in three subjects more than one latin square is possible. For example the following is an alternative:

$$
\begin{array}{ccc}
A & C & B \\
C & B & A \\
B & A & C
\end{array}
$$

As the number of treatments and subjects increases, so the possible order of treatments increases, and the actual latin square used in any one study is decided by randomisation techniques which are best employed with the help of a statistician.

Among the factors that influence a patient's response to drugs are age, sex, duration and severity of the condition which is being treated. In order to obtain a valid comparison of the activities of various preparations, therefore, it is desirable to match patients within treatment groups for these various factors. This may prove impossible, however, particularly if the condition is relatively uncommon. As many factors as possible should be matched, and the limitations imposed by others which are unmatched should be recognised.

Under this heading may be mentioned variations in drug response due to differences in patients' weight. In animal experiments it is usual to give the dose of a drug on the basis of body weight, but in therapeutic practice in man this is seldom done except where toxicity is high, and dose-related. In fixed-dose studies blood and tissue levels of a drug tend to be higher in lighter subjects, and this may obviously produce differences in therapeutic response and toxicity. It may be wise, therefore, either to match patients for weight as well as the other factors mentioned, or to relate the dose to the patient's weight. In practice, however, these precautions are seldom taken, and this may account in part for the wide variations in response which are often reported in trials of centrally acting drugs. One way of monitoring such variations would be to determine the blood levels of the preparations used.

One way of avoiding too great a disparity between two or more treatment groups is to use stratified randomisation. In this approach patients are categorised according to factors which are thought to be relevant to outcome, such as the severity of the condition, or the duration of the particular episode in question. The end result of such a procedure is to produce two groups of patients which are comparable as far as the numbers of severely ill and less severely ill are concerned, and for longer duration and shorter duration of illness.

Another way of achieving a similar result is to apply the minimisation method, the details of which can be found in more specialised textbooks.

3 *Ethical considerations* The ethical issues raised by a proposed clinical trial need to be considered from the outset. The Declaration of Helsinki issued by the World Medical Association in 1960 and revised in 1975 set out the ethical principles to be observed. Two injunctions are of particular importance:

> Every biomedical research project should be preceded by careful assessment of predictable risks in comparison with foreseeable benefits to the subject or others. Concern for the interest of the subject must always prevail over the interests of science and society.

> In any research on human beings, each potential subject must be adequately informed of the aims, methods, anticipated benefits and potential hazards of the study and the discomfort it may entail. He or she should be informed that he or she is at liberty to abstain from participation in the study and that he or she is free to withdraw his or her consent to participation at any time. The doctor should then obtain the subject's freely-given informed consent, preferably in writing.

It will be readily apparent that these principles raise particular problems when applied to the study of psychotropic drugs in psychiatric patients. Informed consent obviously requires the patient having the ability to understand what is intended and the ability to form a reasoned judgment on the merits of the proposal. The ability to understand what is intended may well be impaired in cases of dementia; if so it is essential to discuss the proposed participation of the subject in the clinical trial with a close relative, and to obtain his or her agreement. The ability to form a reasoned judgment on the merits of the proposed study can be affected by delusory ideas, particularly by delusions of persecution as occur in paranoid states, by delusions of unworthiness occuring in severe depressive illnesses, and by grandiose overconfidence as seen in mania. Here too a close relative should be consulted, and it is often advisable to discuss the question of informed consent with a senior colleague as well. In most countries, it is now mandatory to have the proposed research project approved by a local ethical committee which will also doubtless be concerned with these issues.

Assessment of unwanted effects

The unwanted effects of any treatment are often referred to as 'side effects'; however, the unwanted effect in one situation may become a desirable clinical action in another; for example, the sedative action of amitriptyline can be bothersome in the mildly depressed patient but very useful in the more severely depressed patient with insomnia.

The presence and severity of unwanted effects can be ascertained by asking the patient about any possible untoward symptoms, by clinical examination, and by laboratory testing.

1 *Rating of subjective symptoms* There are two basic approaches to the determination of subjective side effects. In one a comprehensive check list of all possible symptoms is completed before starting the drug trial and at various times during its course. In this way it is hoped to allow for the influence of the illness itself on these symptoms. However, many such symptoms occur both as a result of the illness and as a consequence of drug treatment; for example, dryness of the mouth due to a reduction in salivary volume, which is frequently associated with depressive illness, is also a commonly reported side effect of many antidepressant drugs. Rating the presence of such a potential side effect before treatment begins may mask the emergence of a true drug-related symptom.

The other approach to the ascertainment of side effects is to ask an open-ended question after treatment has begun, such as 'Have you noticed that the treatment is affecting you in any way?' This approach minimises the effects of patient expectation in the expression of subjectively experienced side effects. In practice a short check list plus one or more open-ended questions is to be preferred.

2 *Clinical examination* Signs of disturbance within the extra-pyramidal system frequently accompany treatment of schizophrenia with antipsychotic drugs (see chapter 6). The evaluation of such drug-related effects is most reliably undertaken using a standardised examination procedure coupled to a well-defined scoring system. A good example of this type of approach is the *Abnormal Involuntary Movement Scale* (AIMS) devised by the US National Institute of Mental Health.

Clinical assessment of extrapyramidal systems may be supplemented by physical measurements with modern equipment. For example, using a piezoelectric accelerometer with computerised power spectral analysis, it has been shown that the onset of clinical signs of extrapyramidal impairment correlates closely with a reduction in the frequency of finger tremor.

3 *Laboratory procedures* Certain unwanted drug effects are due to alteration in physiological function and can thus be measured using appropriate techniques such as have already been discussed in the section of psychophysiological tests.

In addition it may be helpful to correlate the onset of unwanted effects with the plasma level of the drug in question. Many drugs produce side effects only when the concentration in the plasma exceeds a certain level; this is particularly true in the case of lithium where close monitoring of lithium plasma levels is essential (see chapter 7).

Statistical analyses

Although statistical analysis of the data obtained occurs at the end of a clinical trial, it is advisable to seek the assistance of a statistician in the planning phase to advise on the number of patients required, randomisation procedures and statistical techniques to be employed.

In the past many drugs have been introduced into clinical

practice on the basis of unqualified clinical judgment on the part of a few investigators who had used the compounds in an open, uncontrolled way. The purpose of the measures already discussed was to eliminate observer and patient bias as far as possible, and the mathematical handling of the results obtained is the climax of this process. Table 6 shows the difference in enthusiasm for new drugs when statistical methods were used rather than conclusions based on the global judgment of patients or doctors.

Statistical methods require numerical values which can be analysed, and this is a major problem with psychotherapeutic agents. Whereas drugs such as diuretics and antihypertensive agents produce changes which can be quantified in terms of urine volume or blood pressure, anxiety and changes of mood cannot be evaluated in this way. The rating scales already described may go part of the way to resolving the problem, but they cannot be said to be entirely satisfactory, as the units used bear no constant mathematical relationship to one another. Nevertheless, where it is possible to obtain numerical values, as, for example, the number of subjects showing improvement, deterioration, or relapse, using an overall assessment, or in specific items on rating scales, then statistical techniques should be used. It is not the purpose of this book to describe them in detail, and readers are referred to specialist books on the subject, some of which are mentioned at the end of the chapter. Although simple tests such as Chi squared, Student's t and ranking methods may be sufficient where large and obvious differences between treatments are seen, more sophisticated methods are available which may show significant differences which are not so readily apparent. Particularly valuable are the multivariate techniques of analysis of variance, covariance and dispersion, which minimise differences in results due to other

Table 6   *Effect of statistical analysis on the outcome of clinical trials*

Basis of conclusion	*Studies reporting less than 70% of patients improving*		*Studies reporting 70% or more of patients improving*	
	no.	%	no.	%
Global judgment	175	(48)	191	(52)
Statistical tests	27	(59)	19	(41)

From *Psychopharmacology Bulletin*, March 1969

factors such as between-subject and between-time variations, so that the between-treatments differences may be more readily seen. Such methods of analysis are very complicated, however, particularly when several symptoms and signs are being assessed, and computer facilities are almost always essential for their use.

Where the results of treatment can only be assessed in terms of global judgment, as for example, whether a patient has improved or not improved, and where there are important ethical or other reasons for discontinuing the trial as soon as a statistically significant result is obtained, the *sequential trial* may be appropriate. This involves making preferences for one form of treatment against another, either within patients or between matched patients, and plotting these on a graph prepared from tables, once the statistical requirements for significance have been decided. When a line of significance is crossed, either for one drug against another, or for no difference between treatments, then the trial can be discontinued. For studies of centrally acting drugs, as for most types of clinical trial, a figure of 5 per cent is usually taken as being significant, so that the chances of obtaining a positive result when in fact it does not exist are less than 5 per cent; equally, the chances of not obtaining a positive result when one really exists are also less than 5 per cent.

Phase IV trials

This term refers to studies carried out after a drug has been on the market. Such studies may take the form of further controlled clinical trials on selected populations. Of greater importance is post-marketing surveillance where a careful watch is maintained, through close monitoring of prescriptions, on any adverse effects which had not been expected on the basis of clinical trials information.

Suggestions for further reading

Behavioural pharmacology

FILE, S. E., 'Animal tests of anxiety', *Recent Advances in Neuropsychopharmacology*, ed. B. August, Pergamon Press, Oxford, 1981, pp. 241–51.

IVERSEN, S. D., and IVERSEN, L. L., *Behavioural Pharmacology*, 2nd edn, Oxford University Press, New York, 1981.

KEEHN, J. D., *Animal Models for Psychiatry*, Routledge & Kegan Paul, London, 1986.

Laboratory testing procedures

HINDMARCH, I., 'Psychomotor function and psychoactive drugs', *British Journal of Clinical Pharmacology*, vol. 10, 1980, pp. 189–209.

ITIL, T. M., 'Psychotropic drugs and the human EEG', in *Electroencephalography*, ed. E. Neidermeyer and F. Lopes da Silva, Urban & Schwarzenberg, Baltimore, 1982, pp. 499–513.

LADER, M., *The Psychophysiology of Mental Illness*, Routledge & Kegan Paul, London, 1975.

NICHOLSON, A. N., 'The significance of impaired performance', in *Medicines and Road Traffic Accidents*, ed. D. Burley and T. Silverstone, International Clinical Psychopharmacology, vol. 3, Suppl. 1, 1988.

TURNER, P., 'Tests of autonomic function in assessing centrally acting drugs', *British Journal of Clinical Pharmacology*, vol. 10, 1980, pp. 93–9.

Clinical ratings

LADER, M., 'The clinical assessment of depression', *British Journal of Clinical Pharmacology*, vol. 11, 1981, pp. 5–14.

LITTLEJOHNS, D. W., and VERE, D. W., 'The clinical assessment of analgesic drugs', *British Journal of Clinical Pharmacology*, vol. 11, 1981, pp. 319–32.

MACKAY, A. V. P., 'Assessment of antipsychotic drugs', *British Journal of Clinical Pharmacology*, vol. 11, 1981, pp. 225–36.

MARSDEN, C. D., and SCHACHTER, M., 'Assessment of extrapyramidal disorders', *British Journal of Clinical Pharmacology*, vol. 11, 1981, pp. 129–51.

MAXWELL, C., 'Sensitivity and accuracy of the visual analogue scale', *British Journal of Clinical Pharmacology*, vol. 6, 1978, pp. 15–24.

NICHOLSON, A. N., 'Visual analogue scales and drug effects in man', *British Journal of Clinical Pharmacology*, vol. 6, 1978, pp. 3–4.

SILVERSTONE, T., and COOKSON, J., 'The biology of mania', in *Recent Advances in Clinical Psychiatry*, vol. 4, ed. K. Granville-Grossman, Churchill Livingstone, Edinburgh, 1982, pp. 201–42.

TRIMBLE, M. R., *New Brain Imaging Techniques and Psychopharmacology*, Oxford University Press, Oxford, 1986.

Clinical trials

HAMILTON, M., *Lectures on the Methodology of Clinical Research*, 2nd edn, Churchill Livingstone, Edinburgh, 1974.

MAXWELL, A. E., *Basic Statistics in Behavioural Research*, Penguin Books, Harmondsworth, 1970.

MAXWELL, C., *Clinical Research for All*, Cambridge Medical Publications, 1973.

POCOCK, S. J., *Clinical Trials*, Wiley, Chichester, 1983.

ROBSON, C., *Experiment, Design and Statistics in Psychiatry*, Penguin Books, Harmondsworth, 1973.

SIEGEL, S., *Non-parametric Statistics for the Behavioural Sciences*, McGraw-Hill, Tokyo, 1956.

Social and psychological aspects of drug treatment

5

We educate our patients and their friends to believe that every or almost every symptom and disease can be benefited by a drug, some ignorant practitioners believe this.

Cabot, 1906

National patterns of psychotropic drug prescribing and attitudes

Although written over eighty years ago, Cabot's caustic observation still has considerable force today; particularly in the case of emotional distress where the number and variety of pharmacological preparations prescribed for the relief of tension and anxiety has increased at a remarkable rate in recent years. For example, in the UK during the ten-year period 1966 to 1975 the number of prescriptions issued by general practitioners for drugs classified by the Department of Health and Social Security as 'Tranquillisers' almost doubled, rising from 13.7 million in 1966 to 24.3 million in 1975; and over the same period the number of prescriptions for non-barbiturate hypnotics trebled. After 1975, however, the increase slowed and recently the number of prescriptions issued for tranquillising drugs has begun to fall (Figure 6).

A similar pattern has been observed in the USA. It has been estimated that approximately 10 per cent of the population in both countries currently take some form of psychotropic medication each day, these drugs accounting for 15–20 per cent of all prescriptions. The cost to the community for such prescriptions is staggering, exceeding £50 million in the UK and $1 billion in the USA.

The greatest proportion of such prescriptions is for drugs of the benzodiazepine type, accounting for over 90 per cent of all antianxiety drug prescriptions in both the UK and the USA. In the

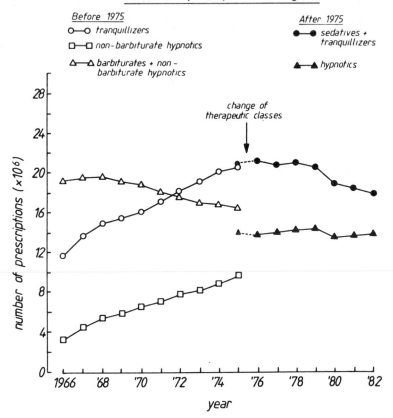

Figure 6   *Number of prescriptions for sedatives, tranquillizers and hypnotics written for NHS non-hospitalized patients in England from 1966 to 1982* [From Edwards, J. G., Cantopher, T., Olivieri, S. *Postgraduate Medical Journal*, 1984, *60* (Suppl 2), 33, by permission]

Boston area it was found that of patients admitted to general medical or surgical wards 15 per cent were taking antianxiety drugs, mainly benzodiazepines; half of them had been taking these drugs for a year or more. A comprehensive general practice survey in the Oxford region revealed that one particular benzodiazepine compound, diazepam, had been described to 6.1 per cent of the total population surveyed during the course of a single year.

Although there has been a general increase in prescriptions for psychotropic drugs throughout the world there are considerable national and even regional variations, not only in the number of prescriptions issued but also in the attitudes to such drugs held by doctors and by potential patients. Comparable surveys of anti-anxiety/sedative drug taking have been undertaken in ten countries under the auspices of the Psychopharmacology Research Branch of the US National Institute of Mental Health.

As can be seen in Table 7, in 1981 the proportion of the population who had taken an antianxiety drug in the previous twelve months ranged from 7.4 per cent in the Netherlands to 17.6 per cent in neighbouring Belgium. The comparable figures for the

Table 7 *Percentage of the adult population who had taken anxiolytic sedative drugs in the previous twelve months*

	Belgium	Denmark	France	Germany	Italy
Percentage who had used such drugs at any time	17.6	11.9	15.9	12.0	11.5
Rank order	1	7	2	6	8
Percentage who had used such drugs for one month or more	11.6	4.4	8.8	4.9	4.7
Rank order	1	7	2	5	6

	Nether-lands	Spain	Sweden	Switzer-land	UK	USA
Percentage who had used such drugs at any time	7.4	14.2	8.6	14.6	11.2	12.9
Rank order	11	4	10	3	9	5
Percentage who had used such drugs for one month or more	3.2	6.6	2.0	4.3	6.7	3.2
Rank order	9	4	11	8	3	9

UK and the USA were 11.2 and 12.9 per cent respectively.

In all eleven countries the number of women prescribed such drugs greatly exceeded the number of men; prescribing was also more common for patients aged over 45 than for younger ones. When we look at the proportion of the population who had taken antianxiety drugs on a regular basis during the year the rank order is rather different; although Belgium and France still come out as the most frequent users of drugs in the long term as well as the short term, longer-term usage was relatively more common in the UK, with the majority of those taking these drugs having taken them regularly for at least a month. Conversely, use in the USA was more short term, the majority there having taken such drugs for less than a month continuously; the same was true for Switzerland. Thus there is not only a variation in the number of patients who are prescribed these drugs, the pattern of use also varies from country to country.

Somewhat surprisingly the national attitudes to antianxiety drugs did not correspond particularly closely to the prescribing pattern; for example, Belgians were among the most antagonistic towards these drugs, yet Belgian doctors prescribed them more frequently than their colleagues in other countries; the Swedes were among the most favourably disposed but ranked low among regular users. In general, patients or potential patients tended to be more conservative in their attitudes towards the value of these compounds than their doctors. The majority of those questioned believed that intrapersonal factors such as will-power and determination were more important than drugs in overcoming life's problems.

Benzodiazepine anxiolytics are prescribed more frequently to women, who receive about 75 per cent of the total prescriptions; women aged 45–64 are prescribed these drugs more often than other age groups. Approximately 20 per cent of those started on a benzodiazepine are likely to be on it six months later; such longer-term drug administration is particularly prevalent in women with additional social problems, and in older patients. These observations assume added importance in the light of the frequency with which physical dependence to benzodiazepines can develop (see chapter 8).

Drug defaulting

If an effective drug is prescribed in the informed opinion that it will ameliorate distressing symptoms, it is obviously equally important that the patient fully understands the directions for taking it and takes it as directed for as long as is considered necessary. While this may seem a naive truism, surveys have shown that many patients, particularly the elderly, have little idea of either the frequency or the number of tablets they should take, or for how long they should go on taking them. Often the prescribing doctor is unaware of his patient's failure to comply with his instructions; this can lead to accumulation of large quantities of potentially dangerous drugs in the households of such patients. An instance of this undesirable state of affairs was provided from a survey of 500 households in a town in the North of England. A total of 43,000 unwanted tablets and capsules were discovered, over a third of which were psychotropic drugs. Extrapolating from this finding to the UK as a whole it was estimated that some 1,250 million unwanted tablets or capsules are likely to be lying in cupboards and medicine cabinets. Apart from the enormous financial waste (well over £10 million) such caches of drugs are obviously a great source of danger to unwary children as well as providing a ready supply to those intent on taking an overdose.

Another cause for concern in this connection is overprescribing, which can arise as a result of the doctor not being aware of the drugs being prescribed elsewhere for a given patient. One possible way of reducing the risk of this occurring is to ask patients routinely to bring all their medicines to every consultation.

One easily remediable cause for non-compliance among patients who are prescribed drugs by their doctor is inadequate instructions being given to the patient. It has been well said: 'In our society better instructions are provided when purchasing a new camera or automobile than when the patient receives a lifesaving antiobiotic or cardiac drug.' Full and detailed instructions are particularly necessary for those of limited intelligence or whose mental powers are failing. This is especially so when more than one drug is prescribed. Visual aids may be of considerable help in imparting the relevant information and the assistance of relatives should be enlisted where possible.

Another reason for patients failing to take their drugs as intended is the development of side effects. There is therefore little point in prescribing large quantities of tablets if the patient is going to stop taking them as soon as an undesirable side effect develops. This is particularly true in the area of psychotropic drugs, the great majority of which can produce such effects. A further cause for stopping is clinical improvement. Most people dislike taking drugs and will stop as soon as they feel well: this can lead to relapse, particularly in patients prescribed drugs for chronic schizophrenia (see chapter 6), or for recurrent affective disorders (see chapter 7). Among schizophrenics prescribed oral medication 32 per cent were found not to be taking any of their oral medication. The introduction of injectable depot pheno-thiazines was intended to improve the high defaulter rate, but even with this type of medication a 27 per cent defaulter rate can occur. Depressed patients attending a hospital out-patient department were no better; 44 per cent were found not to be taking their antidepressant medication – even though a considerable number of them had insisted they were doing so. The picture in general practice is more variable; it depends partly on the doctor–patient relationship and partly on the condition being treated.

It might be thought that the problem of drug defaulting and non-compliance is largely limited to patients who are not resident in hospital. Far from it, careful screening using chromatographic analysis of urine samples has revealed that a considerable proportion, up to 19 per cent in one study, of psychiatric in-patients are not taking their drugs regularly even though they are issued to them by the nursing staff at appropriate times throughout the day.

Lest such findings be thought to be due to vagaries peculiar to psychiatric patients, it should be pointed out that some 50 per cent of patients suffering from rheumatoid arthritis also failed to observe instructions, as did a high proportion of tuberculous patients on anti-tuberculous medication.

Non-pharmacological factors in drug response

Doctor–patient relationship

The doctor–patient relationship not only influences tablet taking but also has a profound effect on the outcome of any course of treatment. First of all, an understanding approach by the doctor will often be sufficient to relieve the patient of his symptoms, particularly where these are the result of worry or tension. In such a situation the benefit attributed to any medication prescribed may be due more to the doctor's manner, and his attitudes towards the drug in question, than to the pharmacological properties of the drug itself. This can lead to an overvaluation of the drug by the doctor and his patient. Even where a true pharmacological effect can be expected this effect may be modified considerably by the doctor–patient relationship. Not unexpectedly, doctors who evince a sceptical attitude towards the drug they are prescribing do not find such drugs nearly as effective as those who prescribe them with enthusiastic optimism. Patients can also influence drug response; any expectations a patient may have about the drug he is receiving can affect the outcome to treatment. Other factors also play a part: males seem to report fewer undesirable side effects than females, and those of lower intelligence appear to do best overall when treated with psychotropic drugs. This latter finding may be related to the placebo effect.

Placebos

A good definition of what placebos are and how they are used has been formulated by Shapiro:

> A placebo is defined as any therapeutic procedure (or that component of a therapeutic procedure) which is given deliberately to have an effect, or which unknowingly has an effect on the patient's symptom, disease or syndrome, but which is objectively without specific activity for the condition treated. The placebo is also used to describe an adequate control in experimental studies. A placebo effect is defined as the changes produced by placebos.

Many authorities have remarked that a placebo effect was the basis of virtually all medication given before Withering used foxglove in dropsy, Sydenham found Cinchona bark effective in malaria, or Lind noted that fresh fruit was specific for scurvy. Eye of newt and leg of toad are, after all, unlikely to have much in the way of specific activity.

Recent critical interest in the placebo effect has been due in great measure to Beecher, an anaesthetist who observed that soldiers wounded in battle during the Second World War required analgesics less often (in 25 per cent of cases) than surgical patients with far less severe trauma, 80 per cent of whom requested analgesics. He found that a good many of these latter responded to placebo, but whether or not this occurred depended on a number of factors:

1 the nature and quantity of the placebo preparation given
2 the situation and manner in which it was prescribed
3 the social and psychological attributes of the recipient
4 the condition being treated.

1 *The nature and quantity of placebo* It has been suggested that the shape, size and colour of a tablet can each influence the placebo reaction. Very small tablets (which are by implication very potent) and very large tablets produce a greater effect than those of more moderate size.

Although normal subjects appear relatively unaffected by the colour of the tablet, psychiatric patients presenting with symptoms of anxiety or depression show a differential response to differently coloured pills. In one intriguing study, anxiety symptoms were found to respond most readily to green, whereas depression responded better to yellow tablets. Red tablets were the least effective in both conditions. As might be expected, the greater number of tablets prescribed, the greater effect within limits; for instance it has been demonstrated that while one 5 mg capsule of amphetamine was superior to a single identical placebo capsule in suppressing subjective hunger, three placebo capsules were better than one active amphetamine capsule.

2 *The situation and manner in which placebo is prescribed* The profound effect of the doctor–patient relationship in treatment has already been emphasised. Nowhere is this more marked than in placebo treatment. A study which illustrates this point well was carried out on patients presenting with gastrointestinal symptoms associated with diagnosed peptic ulcers. When patients were prescribed a placebo by a *doctor* who told them that they were getting a new medicine which would bring undoubted relief, 70 per cent of the patients reported definite symptomatic improvement; when prescribed a placebo by a *nurse* who informed them that they

were receiving an experimental treatment of unknown efficacy, only 25 per cent benefited. Even the most subtle cues can influence a placebo response. Hidden injection of an inert vehicle by a nurse decreased post-operative pain as much as open injection, whereas machine injection did not. This suggests that hidden injection of a placebo may be accompanied by unintentional cues that elicit a placebo response. In post-experiment interviews patients were unable to identify such cues.

3 *The social and psychological attributes of the recipient* Although the factors discussed above play a large part in determining the strength of the placebo effect some people appear more likely to react to placebo medication than others. As it would be clinically helpful if such placebo reactors (or responders) could be readily identified many attempts have been made to describe the characteristics which distinguish them from non-reactors. Unfortunately, the findings do not really allow of a clear-cut definition of the placebo reactor. Nevertheless, there appears to be general agreement that the placebo reactor tends to be found more often among younger patients, particularly those of lower intelligence. There is no consistent sex difference, although some investigators have observed more frequent placebo responses in women. Most observers have remarked on the sociability and the apparent desire to please exhibited by the placebo reactor, and a relatively high level of anxiety has also been noted. Although perhaps more anxious in the treatment situation than non-reactors, the placebo reactors do not show widespread neurotic traits and are usually of a stable, rather outgoing personality. It is particularly important to recognise the corollary of this, namely that a patient who is demanding in seeking attention, or particularly complaining, is unlikely to be a placebo reactor, and is thus unlikely to respond to inert medication.

4 *Condition being treated* From studies on the effect of analgesics and placebos on post-operative pain Beecher and Lasagna concluded that placebos are most effective in acute severe stressful situations, being of considerable benefit in post-operative pain, with some 30 per cent of patients noting relief. They have also been shown to produce symptomatic relief in other acute conditions, including headache, motion sickness, coryza, angina and anxiety.

5 *Mode of action* If placebos acted purely by suggestion then hysterical conversion symptoms might be expected to improve rapidly, but this is one condition where they have proved relatively ineffective. Comparing the effects of repeated placebo administration to those of repeated aspirin administration in a large group of women in labour, Lasagna and his colleagues observed that the time course of efficacy was very similar in both aspirin and placebo; the placebo response was by no means 'all or none'. Similarly the placebo response may persist during the course of several week's medication whereas a suggestion response usually disappears within a few days.

Two observations which highlight the complex interaction between patient, the clinical staff and the treatment procedure are: (1) Morphine addicts, given saline injections instead of morphine, reported no withdrawal symptoms until the saline injections were stopped. (2) The substitution of placebo for active medication, without either patients or ward staff being aware of the substitution, in a ward of chronic schizophrenic patients led to no deterioration in behaviour in the majority, and only 29 per cent relapsed; however, when the placebo was stopped and no tablets at all were given the relapse rate immediately increased to 85 per cent. The finding that the placebo response to painful stimuli can be modified by the opiate receptor blocking drug naloxone has raised the possibility that the placebo response may be mediated through the release of endogenous opiates.

6 *Side effects of placebo* In many placebo studies subjective reports of untoward effects often appear, with the following being the most frequent: *sleepiness, dryness of the mouth, headache* and *nausea*. It is obviously necessary to exclude placebo effects as a cause of such symptoms.

Often this may be difficult, as, for instance, when drowsiness follows administration of anxiolytic sedatives, or dryness of the mouth follows treatment with antidepressant drugs.

Occasionally, severe placebo reactions occur; widespread dermatitis, and angioneurotic oedema have been reported. Not only adverse reactions but true dependence to placebo have been noted on at least one occasion with the patient showing all the characteristics of the dependency state, including withdrawal symptoms.

7 *Use of placebo*   A placebo may be given wittingly to a patient by a doctor in the hope that it might improve the patient's symptoms and in the knowledge that it is unlikely to make him worse. Few doctors appear to prescribe known inert substances in this manner nowadays, and with the increasing understanding of the psychological factors underlying many symptoms, the indications for such an approach are becoming fewer.

Much more frequently doctors prescribe medicines of doubtful efficacy, whose therapeutic effect is largely, if not entirely, dependent on a placebo response, in the mistaken belief that the drugs given have a definite specific pharmacological action. Although in many cases this belief is not very firmly held, the mere fact of prescribing relieves both patient and doctor – something is being done.

Drugs and driving

All centrally acting drugs, if the dose is high enough, have a profound effect on motor skills and reaction time, as well as on the cerebral mechanisms underlying such functions as perception, anticipation and judgment of distance and speed. All these factors are obviously critical in handling complex machinery or driving, where any impairment may well lead to a serious accident. In spite of the considerable potential risk attached to driving while taking psychotropic drugs, relatively little information is available on the subject. This is surprising in view of the ever increasing number of centrally acting drugs prescribed and the equally expanding volume of traffic on the roads, with a likelihood that a substantial proportion of the driving population must at some time be driving under the influence of a psychotropic drug. According to one estimate the incidence of regular use of psychotropic drugs (mainly antianxiety compounds) among drivers is 2–4 per cent. This figure has been substantiated by the findings in two Scandinavian studies, one from Norway, the other from Finland, in which diazepam, the most commonly prescribed antianxiety drug, was detected in 2 per cent of a control sample of drivers not involved in road traffic accidents (RTA).

As far as accidents are concerned, it would appear from a survey undertaken in England that there is a greater chance of drivers who have been involved in a serious RTA having been described an antianxiety drug in the period immediately preceding their accident. Furthermore, a detailed examination by the UK Transport and Road Research Laboratory of more than 2,000 RTA over a four-year period indicated that 4 per cent of the drivers judged to have been at fault were considered to have been impaired by drugs other than alcohol; this was particularly true for those whose accidents were due to loss of control of their vehicle.

Where blood levels of antianxiety drugs such as diazepam have been measured in drivers involved in RTA and compared to control populations, more RTA victims have had detectable levels of diazepam than the matched controls. In a Norwegian study the proportion of drivers with diazepam in the blood was 20 per cent of the RTA victims who had been admitted to hospital, compared to 2 per cent attending the same hospital for non-RTA-related reasons. An even more tightly controlled investigation was carried out in Finland, in which drivers admitted to hospital after an RTA were compared to control subjects who were matched in terms of having driven in the same area on the same day of the week at the same time of day. In this study, there was a similar difference between RTA victims and control drivers although the magnitude of the difference was less striking: 5 per cent of the drivers who had been in an RTA had diazepam detected in their blood, compared to 1.7 per cent of the control population.

Although such statistics provide sufficient cause for concern, there remains the possibility that some drivers, particularly the very anxious, actually drive better when taking moderate doses of anxiolytic sedatives. What we need to know is whether psychotropic drugs when given to patients in clinical dosage significantly impair their driving behaviour, and whether RTA are more common among patients taking these drugs than among patients with similar presenting symptoms who have not been taking medication. Unfortunately there is no evidence available on these points; the experimental work that has been done on the effects of anxiolytic sedatives on driving has largely been restricted to normal subjects. Furthermore, most investigations have been limited to measuring the effects of drugs on psychomotor tasks in the laboratory, or driving simulators; these can only provide pointers to the likely effects of drugs on driving, as they bear little relationship to actually driving a car in traffic, which is an extremely complex operation involving attention, perception, motor skills, motivation, and social attitudes. However there have been a few trials of drugs on driving a car in restricted traffic-free areas; the findings have been somewhat equivocal but, in general, there appears to be little impairment of car driving by experienced drivers after ingestion of therapeutic doses of anxiolytic sedatives. Alcohol, on the other hand, significantly impairs driving skills under these conditions, and the combination of psychotropic drugs with alcohol can be particularly dangerous.

Until more is known about the effects that centrally acting drugs have on the driving abilities of patients, the very least that every doctor should do is to warn his patients that their driving might be affected, and urge them to be ultra-cautious, even to the point of not driving, particularly during the first few days of medication, when the unwanted effects are most pronounced; they should also be told firmly to avoid alcohol before driving and to stop driving if they feel at all unwell during a journey.

Suggestions for further reading

National patterns of psychotropic drug prescribing and attitudes

BALTER, M. B., MANNHEIMER, D. I., MELLINGER, G. D., and UHLENHUTH, E. H., 'A cross-national comparison of antianxiety/sedative drugs use', *Current Medical Research and Opinion*, vol. 118, Supplement 4, 1985, pp. 5–20.

CLARE, A., 'Anxiolytics in society', in *Psychopharmacology: Recent Advances and Future Prospects*, ed. S. Iversen, Oxford University Press, Oxford, 1985, pp. 65–74.

DUNLOP, D., 'Abuse of drugs by the public and by doctors', *British Medical Bulletin*, vol. 26, 1970, pp. 236–9.

GREENBLATT, D. J., SHADER, R. I., and KOCH-WESER, J., 'Psychotropic drug use in the Boston area', *Archives of General Psychiatry*, vol. 32, 1975, pp. 518–21.

KING, D. J., GRIFFITHS, K., REILLY, P. M., and MERRETT, J. D., 'Psychotropic drug use in Northern Ireland 1966–80', *Psychological Medicine*, vol. 12, 1982, pp. 819–33.

MANNHEIMER, D. I., DAVIDSON, S., BALTER, M. B., MELLINGER, G. D., CISIN, I. H., and PARRY, H. J., 'Popular attitudes and beliefs about tranquillisers', *American Journal of Psychiatry*, vol. 130, 1973, pp. 1246–53.

MELLINGER, G. D., and BALTER, M. B., 'Prevalence and patterns of use of psychotherapeutic drugs', in *Epidemiological Impact of Psychotropic Drugs*, ed. G. Tognoni, C. Bellantuono and M. Lader, Elsevier, Amsterdam, 1981, pp. 117–35.

PARISH, P. A., WILLIAMS, W. M., and ELMES, P. C., 'The medical use of

97

psychotropic drugs', *Journal of the Royal College of General Practitioners*, vol. 23, Supplement no. 2, 1973.

SKEGG, D. C. G., DOLL, R, and PERRY, J., 'Use of medicines in general practice', *British Medical Journal*, vol. 1, 1977, pp. 1561–3.

WILKS, J. M., 'The use of psychotropic drugs in general practice', *Journal of the Royal College of General Practitioners*, vol. 25, 1975, pp. 731–44.

WILLIAMS, P., 'Factors influencing the duration of treatment with psychotropic drugs in general practice', *Psychological Medicine*, vol. 13, 1983, pp. 623–33.

Drug defaulting

BALLINGER, B. R., SIMPSON, E., and STEWART, M. J., 'An evaluation of a drug administration system in a psychiatric hospital', *British Journal of Psychiatry*, vol. 125, 1974, pp. 202–7.

BLACKWELL, B., 'Treatment adherence', *British Journal of Psychiatry*, vol. 129, 1976, pp. 513–31.

HARE, E. H., and WILCOX, D. R. C., 'Do psychiatric in-patients take their pills?' *British Journal of Psychiatry*, vol. 113, 1967, pp. 1435–9.

JOHNSON, D. A. W., and FREEMAN, H., 'Drug defaulting by patients on long-acting phenothiazines', *Psychological Medicine*, vol. 3, 1973, pp. 115–19.

PORTER, A. M. W., 'Drug defaulting in general practice', *British Medical Journal*, vol. 1, 1969, pp. 218–22.

PRICE, D., COOKE, J., SINGLETON, S., and FEELY, M., 'Doctor unawareness of the drugs their patients are taking: a major cause of overprescribing?' *British Medical Journal*, vol. 292, 1986, pp. 99–100.

Non-pharmacological factors in drug response

BEECHER, H. K., 'The powerful placebo', *Journal of the American Medical Association*, vol. 159, 1955, pp. 1602–6.

BLACK, A. A., 'Factors predisposing to a placebo response in new out-patients with anxiety states', *British Journal of Psychiatry*, vol. 112, 1966, pp. 557–67.

HESSBACHER, P. T., RICKELS, K., GORDON, P. E., GRAY, B., MECKELNBURG, R.,, WELSE, C. C., and VENDERVORT, W. J., 'Setting, patient and doctor effects on drug response in neurotic patients', *Psychopharmacologia*, vol. 18, 1970, pp. 180–208.

HUSSAIN, M. Z., 'Effect of shape of medication in treatment of anxiety states', *British Journal of Psychiatry*, vol. 120, 1972, pp. 507–9.

LASAGNA, L., LATIES, V. G., and DOHAN, J. L., 'Further studies on the "pharmacology" of placebo and administration', *Journal of General Psychiatry*, vol. 20, 1966, pp. 84–8.

LEVINE, J. D., and GORDON, N. C., 'Influence of the method of drug administration on analgesic response', *Nature*, vol. 312, 1985, pp. 755–6.

LOWINGER, P., and DOBIE, S., 'What makes the placebo work?' *Archives of General Psychiatry*, vol. 20, 1969, pp. 84–8.

SCHAPIRA, K., MCCLELLAND, H. A., GRIFFITHS, N. R., and NEWELL, D. J., 'Study on the effects of tablet colour in the treatment of anxiety states', *British Medical Journal*, vol. 2, 1970, pp. 446–9.

Drugs and driving

ASHWORTH, B. M., 'Drugs and driving', *British Journal of Hospital Medicine*, vol. 13, 1975, pp. 201–4.

BETTS, T. A., CLAYTON, A. B., and MACKAY, G. M., 'Effects of four commonly used tranquillisers on low-speed driving performance tests', *British Medical Journal*, vol. 4, 1972, pp. 580–4.

BØ, O., HAFFNER, J. F. W., LANGARD, O., TRUMPTY, J. H., BREDESEN, J. E., and LUNDE, P. K. M., 'Ethanol and diazepam as causative agents in road accidents', in *Alcohol, Drugs and Traffic Safety*, ed. S. Israelstam and S. Lambert, Addiction Research Foundation, Toronto, 1976.

BURLEY, D., and SILVERSTONE, T., *Medicines and Road Traffic Accidents*, International Clinical Psychopharmacology, vol. 3, Supplement 1, 1988.

HONKANEN, R., ERTAMA, L., LINNOILA, M., ALHA, A., LUKKARI, I., KARLSSON, M., KIVILUOTO, O., and PURO, M., 'Role of drugs in traffic accidents', *British Medical Journal*, vol. 281, 1980, pp. 1309–12.

SEPPALA, T., LINNOILA, M., ELONEN, E., MATTILA, M. J., and MAKI, M., 'Effect of tricyclic anti-depressants and alcohol on psychomotor skills relating to driving', *Clinical Pharmacology and Therapeutics*, vol. 17, 1974, pp. 451–4.

SILVERSTONE, T., 'Drugs and driving', *British Journal of Clinical Pharmacology*, vol. 1, 1974, pp. 451–4.

SKEGGS, D. C. G., RICHARDS, S. M., and DOLL, R., 'Minor tranquillisers and road accidents', *British Medical Journal*, vol. 1, 1979, pp. 917–19.

Clinical applications

Part **II**

Schizophrenia

6

Introduction

Schizophrenia, a condition which is likely to afflict up to 1 per cent of the population, remains one of the least understood conditions in medical practice. In spite of years of painstaking research by teams of highly competent investigators in centres all over the world, disappointingly little is known of its basic underlying pathology, or of its aetiology. Probably the most significant barrier to advancement is the practical and ethical problem of examining the human brain directly. The biochemical and physiological changes within the depths of the brain, which probably underlie the strange and bewildering array of symptoms characteristic of this illness, remain largely inaccessible to direct examination. Recently, however, a number of techniques have become available which allow visualisation of the intact human brain, and an assessment of its functional activities. These include computerised assisted tomography (CAT scan); nuclear magnetic resonance (NMR); electroencephalographic mapping and positron emission tomography (PET) (see chapter 4). The application of these techniques has revealed that there is an increase in the size of the cerebral ventricles of some schizophrenics which is thought to be secondary to a reduction in the size of certain limbic structures, particularly those in the left side of the brain. EEG and PET scan findings similarly suggest a reduction in the functional activity of these areas.

Genetic evidence suggests that some patients become ill as a result of a strong genetically determined predisposition to the illness whereas others who are less genetically predisposed only develop schizophrenia as a result of environmental influences. Such influences might include birth trauma or neonatal viral infection.

Psychopathology

It is perhaps not surprising that no single theory of schizophrenia has obtained universal acceptance when one considers that there are a number of subtypes of the illness, and that its manifestations can vary considerably from patient to patient depending on the subtype present, the cultural background and the pre-morbid personality. There are four main areas of psychological function which may be disturbed in schizophrenia, and correspondingly four varieties of the condition. The areas of malfunction involve perception, thought processes, emotional responsiveness, and motor activity.

Perceptual disorders

The most frequent of the perceptual disorders are auditory hallucinations (hearing voices). Patients can usually hear involved conversations between two or more voices (phonemes) which frequently make disparaging references to the patient, referring to him in the third person. Sometimes the voices will give the patient orders thereby producing unpredictable behaviour. Other hallucinations (i.e. perceptions without stimuli) can occur, such as sensations of electricity in the skin (tactile hallucinations) and strange smells or tastes (olfactory and gustatory hallucinations). Visual hallucinations are rare in schizophrenia, although characteristic of hallucinogenic drug-induced states. Auditory hallucinations also occur in chronic alcohol poisoning and acute amphetamine intoxication, implying a definite organic basis for their origin.

Thought disorder

Many schizophrenic patients, although not lacking in intelligence, are unable to put their thoughts together in a comprehensible fashion. This leads to a failure by the observer to grasp exactly what it is the patient is saying although the individual words and phrases appear to be quite normal. It is this peculiar lack of understandability of the train of thought which, when present, is pathognomonic of schizophrenia. Thought disorder of the schizophrenic type does not occur in any other mental illness and is not produced by any of the hallucinogenic drugs. Thus, hypotheses of schizophrenia based solely on a hallucinogenic drug model are unlikely to provide a complete answer to the problem of understanding the biochemical basis of the illness.

As well as having a disordered way of thinking (disorder of form), schizophrenia patients frequently believe quite irrationally that they are being persecuted, pursued or spied upon (paranoid delusions). Such delusions (or disorders of content) may exist without any disorder of form being present. Paranoid delusions, like auditory hallucinations, may also occur in amphetamine intoxication and in acute confusional states (see chapter 9). Other disorders of thought content include ideas that messages are being given to the patient on the radio or in the newspapers (ideas of reference) and the feeling that he is being controlled by an outside influence (passivity feelings).

Emotional disturbance

Characteristically, schizophrenic patients appear lacking in emotional responsiveness, presenting a blank, disinterested facial appearance (emotional 'flattening'); sometimes they may respond quite unexpectedly by laughing in the wrong place, or giggling to themselves (incongruity of affect); both these phenomena are particularly prevalent in the hebephrenic and simple forms of schizophrenia.

Motor behaviour

Certain patients gradually become less and less active, lapsing eventually into an apparently stuporous state (catatonia). This state may be interrupted by an outburst of violent activity (catatonic excitement) which ends as suddenly as it begins. Although extreme catatonia is now rare, less severe forms of inactivity and lack of drive are not uncommon.

Types of schizophrenia

Schizophrenia has been classified largely on the basis of the predominant symptoms or group of symptoms present. Whether or not the different types each have different aetiology and pathogenesis is not known.

1 *Paranoid schizophrenia* This is usually of acute onset and is the most common form in the elderly. Auditory hallucinations and paranoid delusions dominate the clinical picture. This form is of good prognosis and the most responsive to neuroleptic drugs.

2 *Hebephrenic schizophrenia* This usually comes on gradually and is of less favourable prognosis. It is more common in adolescents and young adults. Incongruity of affect and schizophrenic thought disorder are the most prominent symptoms.

3 *Catatonic schizophrenia* This is the least common, usually having an acute onset in adolescence, and is characterised by catatonic motor symptoms (see above) with underlying thought disorder and delusions.

4 *Simple schizophrenia* This manifests as a gradual withdrawal from all social activity and a corresponding lack of motivation and drive. Flattening of affect is a feature, and thought disorder may be present.

An alternative approach to the classification of schizophrenia has recently been suggested. Patients who exhibit more positive symptoms, such as hallucinations, delusions and thought disorder, are categorised as having a Type I syndrome, whereas those whose symptoms are of a more negative kind, such as emotional flattening, lack of volitional drive and reduction in motor activity, are categorised as having a Type II syndrome. In general the Type II syndrome usually succeeds the Type I syndrome, but can arise *de novo* as is thought to happen in cases of simple schizophrenia. Although the two syndromes are not completely mutually exclusive, patients who exhibit features of Type II class are more likely to reveal significant cognitive impairment in psychological testing and to show abnormalities on CAT scan, such as dilation of the cerebral ventricles.

Biochemical theories of schizophrenia

Although there is no certainty regarding the biochemical basis of schizophrenia, a number of theories have been put forward: of these the most widely accepted is the dopamine hypothesis.

Dopamine hypothesis

An abnormality of the dopamine (DA) pathways within the brain has been implicated as a pathogenic factor in schizophrenia on the basis of a number of pharmacological observations.

(i) All known effective antipsychotic compounds block dopamine receptors, both *in vivo* and *in vitro*.

(ii) The degree of binding to DA receptors by a wide range of antipsychotic drugs, as measured by the displacement of tritiated spiroperidol bound to DA receptors in a preparation of rat caudate membranes, corresponds to their relative clinical potency.

(iii) All the drugs effective in the treatment of schizophrenia invariably raise serum prolactin levels. As the release of prolactin from the pituitary is under tonic dopaminergic inhibition, any reduction in such inhibition, as for example occurs with blockade of DA receptors, results in an increase in prolactin release. The measurement of serum prolactin can provide a clinically useful method for determining whether or not a given dose of a drug is exercising a pharmacological effect in a particular patient, although there is only a tenuous relationship between the degree of prolactin rise and clinical efficacy (see below).

(iv) Amphetamine, which in high dosage can produce a psychosis closely resembling paranoid schizophrenia in normal subjects, and exacerbate paranoid symptoms in patients with pre-existing schizophrenia, is thought to act within the CNS by releasing DA and noradrenaline from nerve terminals. In keeping with this view are the findings that the concentration of the metabolite of DA, homovanillic acid (HVA) in the cerebrospinal fluid of human subjects rises after the administration of amphetamine, and the level of prolactin in the blood falls. Furthermore, amphetamine-related paranoid symptoms are ameliorated by the same antipsychotic drugs which improve spontaneously occurring schizophrenia.

(v) Of the two optical isomers of flupenthixol, the *cis* and the *trans* forms, it is only the *cis* isomer, which blocks DA receptors *in vitro*, which has any significant antipsychotic action in schizophrenic patients, further supporting the view that clinical efficacy depends on central DA receptor blockade.

(vi) Examination of DA receptor density in brains (especially of D_2 receptors) obtained from schizophrenic patients after death has revealed an increase in number of DA receptors in certain major dopaminergic areas of the brain (caudate nucleus, putamen and nucleus accumbens). Although prolonged drug treatment will produce similar changes in receptor density, the finding of increased tritiated spiroperidol binding, which reflects receptor density, has also been found in patients who were believed never to have received any treatment with antipsychotic drugs. It is also of considerable interest that such increase in receptor density was found to a greater degree in those patients who, during life, exhibited the so-called positive symptoms of schizophrenia (delusions, hallucinations and thought disorder) as compared to those who were handicapped by more negative symptoms (emotional flattening, lack of volitional drive and reduction in motor activity). The increase in receptors in the brain of schizophrenics appears specific to D_2 receptors as none of the other neurotransmitter systems when tested with appropriate ligands shows a similar increase in receptor number.

In spite of the convincing array of evidence in support of the DA hypothesis quoted above it would be an oversimplification to suggest that schizophrenia in all its varied forms is but a reflection of a generalised overactivity within DA pathways, or of a supersensitivity of DA receptors throughout the brain. Examination of the CSF of schizophrenic patients has failed to reveal any significant increase in the metabolites of DA; this would argue against any generalised increase of DA in the acute condition.

It should be remembered (see chapter 2) that there are at least five distinct DA pathways within the brain: the nigro-striatal which is concerned with motor coordination and which is affected by Parkinson's disease; the medullary pathway which is possibly identical with the vomiting centre; the hypothalamic–pituitary pathway which affects the release of the hormone prolactin from the pituitary (DA is thought to be an inhibitor of prolactin release by the pituitary); the mesolimbic pathway, which has extensions to the cortex. It is this mesolimbic pathway which is believed to be the one most likely to be involved in schizophrenia.

Other evidence against a general abnormality of brain DA being a causal feature in schizophrenia is the finding that prolactin levels are not lowered in patients with the illness as would be expected if DA were non-specifically increased throughout the CNS; furthermore, parkinsonism, which is a reflection of DA insufficiency within the nigro-striatal system, can coexist with schizophrenia. Thus schizophrenia can hardly be due to a generalised excess DA activity, although it does not rule out a more localised overactivity of DA, perhaps in the mesolimbic system. In keeping with such a view is the observation that the relative potency of antipsychotics as antipsychotic agents in man is closely reflected by their relative potency as DA receptor blockers in the limbic system, but not in the nigro-striatal system of laboratory animals. It would appear that abnormality of DA, either in terms of metabolism, or release, or of the receptors within the mesolimbic system of the brain, is associated with schizophrenia; lesions of this system, such as occur in some cases of temporary lope epilepsy, can lead to a syndrome resembling schizophrenia. But before we can assume that, because antipsychotics act as DA receptor blockers, schizophrenia is due to overactivity in one or more DA systems within the brain, we must consider other alternatives. Schizophrenia may be the result of an imbalance between more than one neurotransmitter system. A hint that this might be so is provided by the finding that physostigmine, a centrally active cholinesterase inhibitor (which leads to excess acetylcholine at the synapse due to reduced breakdown by cholinesterase), can protect against methylphenidate-induced exacerbation of schizophrenia, without being effective against the underlying condition. It may be that the DA mesolimbic pathway is involved in arousal which in turn affects some other, as yet unknown, part of the brain in which the primary lesion lies. If this were true the action of the antipsychotics would be to reduce central arousal, thereby secondarily affecting this, as yet hypothetical, primary system; these drugs would not, however, directly affect the fundamental lesion. Such a view would be consistent with the failure of a proportion of patients with schizophrenia to improve on medication with antipsychotic drugs and it would explain the lag observed between the action of an antipsychotic drug in increasing the level of serum prolactin which begins within 24 hours of starting treatment, and the effects on the clinical symptoms of schizophrenia which may not become apparent for some days, or even weeks.

Other possible imbalances between neurotransmitters have been suggested: these include an increase in DA relative to NA, and an increase of DA relative to 5-hydroxytryptamine (5–HT). This latter suggestion would also involve the concept of arousal, as

5–HT is generally believed to be concerned in the regulation of sleep and waking; with lowered 5–HT reducing sleep and increasing arousal. Thus elevation of DA activity and reduction of 5–HT activity could act synergistically to increase arousal and thereby exacerbate the underlying schizophrenic syndrome.

We would conclude that, while it would appear that DA is involved in the pathogenesis of schizophrenia in some way in some patients, the exact mechanism underlying such involvement is, as yet, undetermined.

Pharmacology of antipsychotic drugs

The antipsychotic drugs used in the treatment of schizophrenia were originally referred to as neuroleptic compounds because of their ability to produce a state of 'neurolepsis' or calm indifference, without loss of consciousness. The antipsychotic drugs are usually classified according to their chemical configuration. The chemical groupings include phenothiazines, thioxanthenes, indole derivatives, butyrophenones, diphenylbutypiperidines and benzamide derivatives.

Phenothiazines

The discovery that the phenothiazine derivative promethazine possesses sedative and antihistamine actively encouraged the synthesis of other compounds in this group. Chlorpromazine, synthesised in 1950, was soon found to have pronounced calmative effects on disturbed psychotic patients. Since then it has come to be the standard compound against which other substances have been compared. Phenothiazines have a large number of pharmacological properties, and minor changes in their molecular structure may profoundly influence their therapeutic activity and the severity of unwanted effects, particularly the incidence of extrapyramidal reactions. All drugs in this group have in common the phenothiazine nucleus shown in the diagram:

Derivatives are usually formed by substitution at positions R_1 and R_2. The side chains at R_1 may be classified into three groups: (i) dimethylaminopropyl (aliphatic) (ii) piperazine (iii) piperidine. The substitutions at R_2 include halogens, methoxy, acetyl, thiomethyl, and other organic radicals. Compounds such as promazine, which is unsubstituted at position R_2, are very much less active pharmacologically than derivatives with chloro- or trifluoromethyl substitutions at that position, such as chlorpromazine or trifluopromazine; this variation in pharmacological effect has been related to the stoichiometric configuration of the molecule; Snyder talks of the compounds being 'sculpted' to fit the DA receptor where they act to block transmission by DA. It also appears that the different substituents on the phenothiazine ring determine the site of action by altering the distribution of the drug, the more potent compounds having substituents which increase their lipid solubility and facilitate their transport into the brain. Their pharmacological actions depend on the electronic nature of the phenothiazine ring and involve electron donation in charge-transfer reactions.

In keeping with Snyder's view is the strikingly close correlation which is found between the relative affinity these drugs have for DA receptors in the brain and their relative clinical potency. This is particularly true for binding to D_2 receptors (see chapter 2); a finding which led to the suggestion that D_2 receptors are relatively more important than the adenylate cyclase-linked D_1 receptors in mediating the clinical effects of antipsychotic drugs.

1 *Neurochemical action*   Phenothiazine compounds act by blocking dopamine receptors in all five dopaminergic systems of the brain. After the postsynaptic DA receptors have been blocked by these drugs there is a feedback mechanism whereby the pre-synaptic neurone releases more DA to overcome the blockade; this in turn increases the production and turnover of DA with a corresponding increase in its metabolites. In fact, the finding of such an increase in the metabolites of dopamine led Carlsson to suggest that phenothiazine drugs might act as DA receptor blockers. Reduction of this compensatory DA synthesis, as occurs after blocking the enzyme tyrosine hydroxylase with alpha-methylparatyrosine, enhances the antipsychotic activity of chlorpromazine, thus confirming that it is DA receptor blockade which is the basis of the therapeutic action of chlorpromazine. The relative potency of the

111

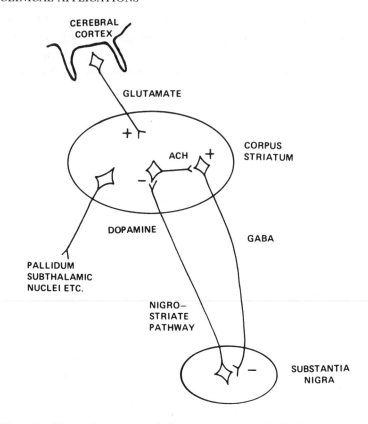

Figure 7   *Scheme of pathways involved in corpus striatum and related structures*

various phenothiazine compounds is not the same at all sites. For example, thioridazine, which has a piperidine side chain, is less effective than a clinically equivalent dose of chlorpromazine, which has an aliphatic side chain, on increasing DA metabolism in the nigro-striatal system; chlorpromazine in turn has less effect than a clinically equivalent dose of fluphenazine, which has a piperazine side chain. This finding is in keeping with the greater tendency of the piperazine phenothiazines to produce extrapyramidal symptoms. Drugs such as thioridazine, which are less likely to produce extrapyramidal symptoms, and which have correspondingly less effect of DA turnover in the striatum, have an in-built anticholinergic action. It is thought that DA neurones in the striatum inhibit acetylcholine neurones, which normally activate gamma amino butyric acid (GABA) neurones. These GABA neurones, in turn, inhibit the DA neurones, see Figure 7. If the action of acetylcholine is blocked at the same time as the DA receptor, then the effects on the motor system are cancelled out, whereas if the acetylcholine system is freed from dopaminergic inhibition, then extrapyramidal symptoms emerge.

In the mesolimbic system, in contrast to what happens in the striatum, the three drugs, thioridazine, chlorpromazine and fluphenazine have similar effects on dopamine turnover when given in clinically equivalent dosage. This finding is consistent with the view that the efficacy of these drugs on schizophrenia is more closely related to a possible action within the mesolimbic system than elsewhere in the brain.

The phenothiazines are potent antiemetic drugs, preventing vomiting produced by other drugs such as apomorphine which stimulate the dopaminergic chemoreceptor trigger zone. An action on neighbouring medullary areas may be responsible for their usefulness in the control of persistent hiccough.

There is at least one other dopaminergic system on which phenothiazines act; that is the hypothalamic pituitary portal pathway which controls the release of prolactin from the pituitary. Dopamine inhibits the release of prolactin so that DA receptor blocking drugs, such as phenothiazines, by preventing this DA mediated inhibition, allow more prolactin to be released into the circulation, thus raising the serum prolactin level. It has recently been found that if the prolactin level rises above 30 ng/ml two hours after the administration of chlorpromazine, extrapyramidal symptoms are likely to follow. Furthermore, there appears to be a significant correlation between the plasma levels of prolactin and of chlorpromazine. A similar relationship between plasma levels of drug, the rise in serum prolactin and the appearance of extrapyramidal symptoms has been observed with haloperidol. Measurement of change in the plasma prolactin level would thus appear to provide a useful index of central dopaminergic blockade as well as affording an indicator of patient compliance (see chapter 5). Although a rise in plasma prolactin occurs during effective treatment with all the currently available antipsychotic drugs, this rise in prolactin often occurs somewhat earlier than the improvement in clinical state. Such a dissociation between the onset of DA receptor blockade in the pituitary (as reflected by the rise in plasma prolactin) and the time of initial clinical improvement has

113

cast some doubt on the theory that the clinical effects of the antipsychotic drugs are *directly* attributable to DA blockade. Furthermore, after stopping treatment with an antipsychotic drug the plasma prolactin level falls to normal within 3 to 4 days without a concomitant recrudescence of psychotic symptoms, which may not occur for several weeks. Only a loose association has been found in a number of studies between the degree of clinical response and the plasma level of the drug being investigated or in the rise of prolactin produced. Raised prolactin levels can produce galactorrhoea in women and gynaecomastia in men. In addition to their DA receptor blocking activity the phenothiazines have a variable anticholinergic activity (see above) and weak to moderate antihistamine and anti-5–HT activity.

2 *Pharmacokinetics* Chlorpromazine, which has been the most widely studied of the phenothiazines, is readily absorbed from the gastrointestinal tract and from intramuscular injection sites, with a peak blood level occurring some 1.5 to 3 hours after oral administration. Sometimes absorption may be poor, with consequently low plasma levels. Distribution within the body is rapid, with the highest concentrations occurring in the lungs, liver, adrenal glands and spleen. Within the brain there would appear to be a selective distribution, with the highest concentration being found in the hypothalamus, basal ganglia, thalamus and hippocampus.

As yet no optimal plasma level for chlorpromazine has been established although the ratio of active metabolites to the more inert ones may be of some importance. Of the metabolites the 7-hydroxy derivative is pharmacologically active whereas the sulphoxide is not; consequently if there is a relatively large proportion of sulphoxide therapeutic response is less. Chlorpromazine has an enzyme-inducing effect which in turn can affect the concentration in the body of other compounds (see chapter 3 for a further discussion of this point).

Chlorpromazine has a plasma half-life of some six hours; however, it can remain bound to the tissues for very long periods, and metabolites may continue to be excreted for up to six months after the patient has stopped taking it.

3 *Interaction with other drugs* Phenothiazines enhance the central depressant effects of many other drugs including barbiturates and alcohol.

While they only possess a weak anticholinergic activity themselves, when combined with an anticholinergic compound prescribed to relieve parkinsonian side effects, an atropine-type psychosis can occur due to the additive atropine-like activity.

Thioxanthenes

The thioxanthene compounds are chemically closely related to the phenothiazines, the nitrogen in the central ring having been replaced by carbon, and they appear to have similar pharmacological effects. Flupenthixol appears to have a mood elevating effect (see chapter 7).

Butyrophenones

Although the butyrophenone compounds are structurally distinct from the phenothiazines they share many of their pharmacological properties. Like the phenothiazines they cause accumulation of O-methylated metabolites of dopamine and noradrenaline within the brain, suggesting that they also block dopamine and noradrenaline receptors, thus causing compensatory activity of central neurones with monoamine transmitter release. In the peripheral autonomic nervous system butyrophenones such as haloperidol and trifluperidol selectively block dopamine receptors in the renal and mesenteric vascular beds, and it may be that a similar selectivity of action occurs in the central nervous system.

The butyrophenones are also potent antiemetic drugs, suppressing activity of the chemoreceptor trigger zone, and they produce extrapyramidal disorders similar to those accompanying phenothiazine medication. They also potentiate the sedative effects of alcohol, analgesics, anaesthetics and barbiturate drugs, and transient orthostatic hypotension can occur, due to peripheral adrenergic receptor blockade.

Diphenylbutylpiperidines

These compounds, derived from the butyrophenones, have a more prolonged duration of action. They would also seem to have a more specific dopamine receptor blocking action. Two members of this group are in clinical use, pimozide, which can be given orally on a daily basis, and fluspiriline, which requires to be administered intramuscularly, a single injection of which has an effective action of one week.

Benzamide derivatives

Sulpiride, a member of this class of compounds (which also includes metoclopramide), has been shown to be effective in the treatment of both acute and chronic schizophrenia. Pharmacologically, sulpiride differs from phenothiazine and butyrophene derivatives in that it has greater relative activity in blocking D_2 receptors as compared to D_1 receptors (see chapter 2). Theoretically this might result in the drug having less tendency to produce unwanted extrapyramidal symptoms (see below). In keeping with this possibility are the findings from two controlled clinical trials in which sulpiride was found to be as effective as chlorpromazine in the management of acute schizophrenia, and trifluoperizine in chronic schizophrenia, with the suggestion that extrapyramidal side effects were less troublesome in the patients receiving sulpiride, although the differences failed to reach statistical significance.

Other drugs

Tetrabenazine is a synthetic benzoquinolizine which retains some of the structural features of reserpine and has an identical pharmacology. It depletes the brain of its monoamine stores and this is probably the basis of its sedative and antipsychotic effects. Mental depression and extrapyramidal reactions commonly occur. Its dopamine depleting property is said to be useful in the management of tardive dyskinesia.

Certain indole derivatives, such as oxypertine and molindone appear to possess antipsychotic properties. Other dibenzyl structures including clozapine and metiapine have similar effects with less tendency to produce parkinsonian symptoms.

Following observations that the beta-adrenoceptor blocking drug propranolol controlled the psychosis in a patient with acute porphyria, several groups of investigators reported marked improvement in some patients with schizophrenia when treated with propranolol in doses considerably higher than those used in cardiovascular disease. In most cases propranolol has been used together with standard phenothiazine antipsychotic drugs, and there is evidence that there may be competition for the same hepatic metabolic pathways leading to increased tissue and blood phenothiazine levels. Studies involving the use of propranolol alone have generally produced unconvincing or negative results, although at least one double-blind controlled study has shown that it was as effective as, if not superior to, thioridazine in patients with chronic schizophrenia. It is uncertain if this action is mediated by beta-adrenoceptor blockade. Propranolol inhibits 5–HT induced hyperactivity in animals and, together with other beta-blockers, inhibits the specific binding of 5–HT to brain synaptosomal membranes. There is, as yet, no good evidence that it is a dopamine-receptor antagonist.

Drug treatment

Acute schizophrenia

An acute schizophrenic episode frequently presents with obvious delusory ideas, accompanied by auditory hallucinations. In addition there may be frank thought disorder with ideas of reference, ideas of influence and passivity feelings. Such a situation, whether arising for the first time, or resulting from a relapse in a patient who has had a similar illness in the past, calls for energetic medication with one of the neuroleptic drugs. This can be done either on an in-patient or an out-patient basis, although generally speaking the majority of patients suffering from acute schizophrenia will require in-patient treatment for a short time, particularly if they are disturbed in their behaviour.

1 *Initial control* Once the diagnosis of acute schizophrenia has been made, the next step is to decide on the choice of medication and the route of administration. If, as is usually the case, there is a certain amount of motor excitement, arising perhaps out of the patient's delusional fears, administration of a neuroleptic with sedative effects would be advisable. A phenothiazine with an aliphatic side chain such as chlorpromazine is particularly suitable. It is difficult to be dogmatic about dosage but the following guidelines are suggested:

(i) In the case of a healthy male patient under the age of sixty, up to 300 mg of the drug may be given as a starting dose. This

117

can be repeated as necessary up to four times in twenty-four hours for the first few days. In most cases it is usually possible to reduce the dosage to between 100 and 200 mg twice to four times daily within a short time. The physician will need to be guided on the one hand by the amount by which disturbed behaviour has been reduced and on the other hand by the degree of somnolence produced by the medication. It may be that the first dose produces so much drowsiness that the dosage can be sharply reduced almost immediately. Sometimes, however, even 300 mg of chlorpromazine proves inadequate to reduce the acute disturbance sufficiently and an even higher dosage may be required. In many cases with frank behaviour disturbance, the oral route is not possible and the drug has to be given intramuscularly, when the dosage should be halved. Intramuscular administration is rarely required after the first 24–48 hours, as by then the patient has usually become sufficiently cooperative to take his drugs by mouth. Because of the smaller volume required to be injected, haloperidol may be considered preferable when parenteral administration is required (see below).

(ii) A healthy woman under the age of sixty should be given up to 200 mg chlorpromazine as a starting dose if given orally, or 100 mg if given by injection, otherwise the initial drug treatment is as outlined for a healthy male.

(iii) A patient who is known to be in frail physical health, or anyone over the age of sixty, should not be given more than 100 mg chlorpromazine in the first instance. Particular care should be taken in patients with cardiovascular abnormalities lest drug-induced hypotension should embarrass their circulation yet further. Similarly those with a known history of liver disease should be treated cautiously as they are often particularly sensitive to the central effects of phenothiazine compounds.

Haloperidol (Haldol, Serenace) may be substituted for chlorpromazine either when an injection is required or when given orally. Haloperidol is approximately ten to twenty times more potent than chlorpromazine, thus for a healthy man the appropriate dose of haloperidol is 30 mg, or 15 mg by injection; for a healthy woman, 20 mg orally or 10 mg by injection; for the frail or elderly, 10 mg orally or 5 mg by injection. It is claimed that haloperidol acts rather more quickly and produces less sedation than chlorpromazine, with less risk of hypotension occurring. Furthermore the rapid intravenous administration of relatively high doses of haloperidol has been recommended as being more effective than the standard regime. Controlled clinical trials have failed to substantiate this.

2 *Amelioration of schizophrenic symptoms* Once control of disturbed behaviour has been achieved the next step is to decide upon the most suitable treatment of the particular symptom complex present in the individual case. The symptoms most responsive to neuroleptic medication are paranoid delusions and auditory hallucinations; thought disorder, apathy and abnormalities of emotional response are less likely to improve so gratifyingly.

There is a bewildering choice of drugs available, all of which have been claimed to be useful in the management of schizophrenia. These include some ten phenothiazine compounds, four thioxanthene derivatives, four butyrophenones and two members of the closely related diphenylbutylpiperidines, at least one substituted benzamide, plus a number of others (see Table 8).

Several well-conducted large-scale clinical trials have failed to reveal any significant differences in overall efficacy between one neuroleptic phenothiazine and another. Furthermore, although it had been suggested that those phenothiazine drugs with piperazine side chains (e.g. trifluoperazine and fluphenazine) were more effective than the aliphatic phenothiazines (e.g. chlorpromazine) in stimulating apathetic schizophrenic patients into activity, the evidence obtained from the clinical trials fails to support this suggestion. Similar claims have been made for sulpiride, the more recently introduced substituted benzamide. Thus far controlled trials have failed to show any difference in the pattern of clinical response between sulpiride and either trifluoperazine or haloperidol.

The choice of drug depends more upon the side effects produced, which vary from drug to drug, and upon the frequency of dosage required.

Chlorpromazine remains the standard medication in schizophrenia against which other treatments must be measured. It has been repeatedly shown to be more effective in schizophrenia than an inert placebo or an anxiolytic sedative such as phenobarbitone. It is also better than the antihistamine compound promethazine from which it was originally derived. With chlorpromazine over 60 per cent of patients with acute schizophrenic symptoms can be expected to improve significantly within a matter of weeks. The dosage of chlorpromazine required to achieve this varies considerably from case to case but is rarely less than 100 mg three times a day and may be as high as 300 mg four times daily. Once a steady state has been achieved it may be possible to reduce the dose by half without a recrudescence of symptoms. The drawbacks of chlorpromazine are its sedative effects and tendency to produce extrapyramidal symptoms (see below), together with the possibility of cholestatic jaundice, although the incidence of this is low. If oversedation proves a problem in management with chlorpromazine then one of the piperazine compounds such as trifluoperazine (Stelazine) 5–10 mg or fluphenazine (Moditen, Prolixin) 2.5–5 mg three times daily may be tried. While they are certainly less sedating, they produce rather more extrapyramidal symptoms (see below). In contrast thioridazine (Melleril), 100–200 mg three times daily is the least likely of all the phenothiazines to cause such unwanted effects, but it, too, has its drawbacks. It is as sedative as chlorpromazine and is rather more likely to produce hypotension. In addition it interferes with ejaculation in men and may consequently prove unacceptable to many male patients if given over a period larger than a month or two. In addition there is the risk of producing retinal pigmentation.

Neither the thioxanthene derivatives nor the butyrophenones appear to have any marked advantage over the phenothiazines in the management of schizophrenia. The newer compounds in the diphenylbutylpiperidine group may prove to be more useful. Pimozide (Orap) has been shown to be as effective as haloperidol in the treatment of acute schizophrenia and appears to be less sedating. It requires only once daily administration at a dose of 4 to 40 mg per day. This is not only an advantage to the nurses in a busy psychiatric ward, but it also means that the prescribed dosage is more likely to be taken by the patient at home if he has to remember to take his pills only once during the day instead of three times. In this connection, however, it has recently been suggested that phenothiazine medication need only be given twice daily at most, once initial control has been obtained. Fluspiriline (Redeptin) reduces the frequency of administration required to weekly, but it has to be given intramuscularly, and this may be less acceptable in some patients.

Following initial encouraging reports that the beta-adrenergic blocking drug propranolol had antipsychotic activity, a number of controlled trials were undertaken of d-l propranolol and one of d-propranolol (the isomer with no beta blocking activity) in schizophrenia. At best only a modest antipsychotic effect was observed when propranolol was given alone. When added to existing treatment with chlorpromazine, propranolol appeared superior to placebo, but this may have been due to a pharmaco-kinetic interaction whereby propranolol increased the bioavail-ability of chlorpromazine.

Despite enthusiastic claims for megavitamin therapy in schizo-phrenia, a carefully conducted large-scale controlled trial failed to substantiate them.

3   *Longer-term medication*   How long should one go on treating an acute episode of schizophrenia? There is no really clear-cut answer possible, for that depends on the presenting illness. If the episode is the first manifestation of schizophrenia in a particular patient of a previously good personality, and if there was no emotional abnormality during the illness, which itself was of acute onset and short duration, then the chances are that longer-term medication will not prove necessary. In one study it was found that among a group of such patients given no further medication after discharge from hospital the relapse rate was just over 25 per cent. When these criteria were not met, the relapse rate without further drug treatment among those who had responded reasonably well to treatment in the acute phase was over 80 per cent. In contrast, long-term treatment in this second group reduced the relapse rate to 33 per cent.

In a more recent placebo controlled study of first episode schizophrenia those with a shorter history of illness prior to admission did better, whatever the follow-up treatment, than those who had been ill for more than six months before their first hospital admission for schizophrenia. However, even in the group with the shorter length of illness over 50 per cent of those on placebo relapsed in the following two years compared to less than 30 per cent of those receiving continued medication with an antipsychotic drug. Of the patients who had been ill for longer, continued medication had a less pronounced effect; while less than 10 per cent of those on placebo remained in remission, almost as few on medication did so. Thus some patients will recover completely from acute schizophrenia and require no further drug treatment for the time being.

As 50 per cent of short-illness patients do well without longer-term drug treatment it is warranted to begin gradually reducing the dose of medication in such patients some six months after complete remission. A close watch must be maintained for the next six months for any sign of relapse; should that happen drug treatment should be restarted as soon as possible and continued for the foreseeable future.

Other patients never fully recover in the sense that they can remain symptom-free without medication. This latter group is often referred to as suffering from chronic schizophrenia, and management of this condition raises problems of its own.

Chronic schizophrenia

If after a first attack of schizophrenia the patient relapses after his medication is stopped then it is likely that he is suffering from the chronic form of the condition and will require continuous medication for years, if not for life. While this need for long-term treatment may well be recognised by the medical advisers concerned with treatment, it is frequently not accepted by the patient. Consequent failure to take the medication leads to recrudescence of symptoms with readmission; in fact the most common cause for readmission to hospital is a relapse following failure to take the drugs prescribed.

As in the case of acute schizophrenia, no one neuroleptic drug stands out from the rest in terms of efficacy, provided the drug is taken. Several investigations have revealed how inconstant and unreliable many patients are in their medication. They stop it either because they feel well and can see no point in continuing, or because the side effects are sufficiently unpleasant to deter them from persevering. Although such behaviour is by no means confined to schizophrenics (see chapter 5), it creates particularly severe management problems in them. What is required is some way of ensuring that schizophrenic patients take their medication for as long as is considered necessary. The introduction of long-acting depot preparations given by intramuscular injection every one to four weeks has gone a long way to meeting this requirement. The more commonly used depot preparations include fluphenazine decanoate (Modecate), flupenthixol decanoate (Depixol) and haloperidol decanoate (Haldol decoanate); others are listed in Table 8. Carefully controlled trials have failed to reveal any significant differences between them in terms of efficacy, drop-out rate or the emergence of depressive symptoms. Haloperidol decanoate does appear to cause less weight gain.

Patients are usually asked to attend special clinics to receive their regular injections. This not only allows an efficient routine to be adopted by the patients and the nursing staff administering the fluphenazine injections, but it makes it easy to spot when a patient fails to attend. In that case he can either be asked to come up for his injection at another time, or, failing that, he can be visited in his home by a nurse who can give him the injection there and then. The adoption of such a treatment programme for patients with chronic schizophrenia discharged into the community has been shown to reduce the relapse rate but by no means abolish it.

The dose of medication should be reviewed at least twice a year and every effort made to reduce it to as low a level as is consistent with the amelioration of symptoms. Pimozide (Orap) in a daily oral dose of 8 mg appears to be at least as effective as regular depot injections of fluphenazine, and more recently it has been shown that giving the drug twice a week is equally effective.

The maintenance therapy of those chronic schizophrenic patients whose symptoms do not remit sufficiently for them to live outside hospital is not so difficult to control and supervise. Here the problem may be one of unnecessarily prolonged medication rather than its absence. These patients remain incapable of leading an independent life in spite of adequate neuroleptic treatment. In many cases stopping their drug does not lead to any deterioration in their condition; on the contrary there may be marked improvement associated with lessening of extrapyramidal symptoms. Even in those patients in whom continued medication is shown to be of benefit, a reduction in dosage may be achieved. Therefore, it is advisable to review regularly the medication of all long-term in-patients receiving continuous neuroleptic therapy.

Therapeutic drug monitoring in schizophrenia

Clinical experience shows that there is a wide interpatient variability in therapeutic response to a given dose of antipsychotic drug. An important contribution to this is a large between-subject variation in steady-state plasma levels achieved after a given dose of drug. It might be anticipated, therefore, that measurement of plasma drug levels could improve patient care by providing guidance on appropriate changes in dose. However, therapeutic plasma levels have not been demonstrated for antipsychotic drugs as they have for others such as lithium, and there is no evidence, therefore, that therapeutic drug monitoring is of value in the management of schizophrenia.

Unwanted effects of neuroleptic drugs

1 *Extrapyramidal symptoms*

These can be considered under four headings.

The first three are relatively acute, they are also clearly dose-dependent and disappear when medication ceases. The fourth group appears often to be irreversible, sometimes even getting worse after neuroleptic treatment has ceased.

Such reactions occur in up to 40 per cent of patients treated with phenothiazines, being more common with those compounds having a piperazine side-chain. They are equally frequent with the other chemical classes of antipsychotic drugs, with the possible exception of the benzamide derivatives. Certain of the antipsychotic drugs which have an intrinsic anticholinergic activity, such as thioridazine and clozapine, are less prone to be associated with extrapyramidal symptoms, but even they are by no means completely free from producing these symptoms.

(a) *Acute dystonia* This is an involuntary contraction of skeletal muscles most frequently occurring in the head and neck, giving rise to what is usually referred to as an oculogyric crisis. It begins with a fixed stare which then gives way to a turning upwards of the eyes, followed by hyperextension of the neck and opening of the mouth. The attack may last several hours before subsiding spontaneously. Dyskinestic reactions can also involve the trunk and limbs, producing grotesque postures and writhing movements which are extremely distressing. They occur in some 2 to 10 per cent of patients treated with antipsychotic drugs, usually appearing within a day or two of starting treatment, being commoner in younger male patients. They are thought to result from an increase in the synthesis and release of DA from pre-synaptic vesicles which occurs as an initial response to the blockade of post-synaptic DA receptors; alternatively such an increase in DA release may be due to an early pre-synaptic DA receptor blockade due to a preferential sensitivity of such receptors for antipsychotic drugs.

Acute dystonic reactions respond best to parenteral procyclidine (Kemedrine) 5–10 mg or biperiden (Akineton) 2–5 mg given either by slow intravenous injection or intramuscularly. Intravenous diazepam at a dose of 10 mg has also been found to be effective.

(b) *Pseudo-parkinsonism* The clinical picture mimics idiopathic parkinsonism very closely, with a stiffening of the limbs, lack of facial expression, a characteristic coarse tremor of the hands and head at rest, plus sialorrhoea and seborrhoea. It may progress to a complete seizing up with a virtual absence of movement. Pseudo-parkinsonism has been observed in 20 to 40 per cent of patients receiving antipsychotic drugs. Typically it begins some 11 to 22 weeks after the start of such treatment, being commoner in older patients, especially elderly females. It is believed to be the direct result of DA receptor blockade within the nigro-striatal system which causes functional impairment within that system (as happens in Parkinson's disease itself, although in that disease the functional impairment is due to degeneration of DA cell bodies in the substantia nigra). The relatively increased risk of pseudo-parkinsonism occurring in the elderly has been attributed to a pre-existing subclinical impairment of the nigro-striatal system associated with aging; this renders them more susceptible to the added effects of DA receptor blockade.

The first step in the management of drug-induced pseudo-parkinsonism and akathisia is to stop the drug temporarily or sharply reduce the dose. Many patients will not deteriorate if their medication stops for a few days, particularly if they have been receiving it for several weeks. This measure, together with the administration of an antiparkinsonian drug is usually sufficient. Of those available benzhexol (Artane) 2–4 mg, procyclidine (Kemedrine) 5–10 mg, orphenadrine (Disipal) 50–100 mg, and methixene (Tremonil) 5–10 mg three times daily would appear to be equally effective; contrary to the situation in idiopathic parkinsonism, levodopa makes schizophrenia patients with phenothiazine-induced parkinsonism worse.

Furthermore, the need for continued antiparkinsonian medication should be reviewed in all patients currently receiving it, as several studies have revealed that in the great majority of patients cessation of such medication does not result in recrudescence of extrapyramidal symptoms. There is also evidence that anticholinergic drugs can reduce the efficacy of antipsychotic drugs and, in the elderly, anticholinergic drugs have been shown to impair memory. Thus there are several good reasons for restricting the long-term prescription of anticholinergic drugs to those patients in whom it has been shown to be definitely required for the amelioration of neuroleptic-induced parkinsonism.

There have been a number of reports describing the abuse of anticholinergic drugs, in both schizophrenic patients and in non-schizophrenics. This is a consequence of the mood-elevating properties which these drugs possess. Excessive consumption can lead to a toxic confusional state with vivid visual hallucinations, which may be followed by prolonged cognitive impairment.

We do not recommend the routine administration of anti-parkinsonian agents to all patients receiving neuroleptics. Not only may they be unnecessary, but also they produce other unwanted effects of their own, particularly anticholinergic symptoms which exacerbate the autonomic actions produced by the phenothiazines themselves and have been implicated in the pathogenesis of tardive dyskinesia.

(c) *Akathisia* This is a condition characterised by motor restlessness, a subjective feeling of tension and an inability to tolerate inactivity which gives rise to restless movement. Milder cases present mainly with subjective feelings of inner restlessness, especially referable to the legs. As the condition progresses motor symptoms become evident. Patients typically rock from foot to foot, or walk on the spot when standing and show a coarse tremor of the feet. They may even feel compelled to get up from their chair and walk about.

Acute akathisia occurs in some 20 per cent of patients receiving antipsychotic drugs, and comes on within the first few weeks of treatment. There is a late-onset variant which may be a harbinger of tardive dyskinesia with which it can coexist. In contrast to acute akathisia which improves when the dose of antipsychotic medication is reduced, chronic akathisia worsens. Acute akathisia is thought to be due to blockade of DA receptors in the mesolimbic and mesocortical dopamine pathways. Anticholinergic drugs are ineffective in the majority of cases. Encouraging reports that propranolol, a beta-adrenergic receptor blocking drug, is effective in relieving symptoms at a dose of 30–80 mg daily have been substantiated by a controlled clinical trial.

2 Tardive dyskinesia

This term relates to a chronic syndrome of hyperkinetic involuntary movements which are most frequently limited to the face, lips, tongue, jaw and neck, but which can involve the trunk, arms and hands. There would appear to be two distinguishable subtypes. The first, and by far the most common, is referred to as the 'bucco-linguo-masticatory' (BLM) syndrome. It ranges from infrequent lateral movements of the jaw together with puckering and pouting of the lips and slight tongue movements which distend the cheek, to a clinical picture dominated by unceasing movements of the lower face associated with frequent mouth opening and protrusion of the tongue. The other subtype includes movements of the whole trunk in which body rocking, shoulder shrugging, back arching and even pelvic gyrations appear, the limbs display choreiform movements and myoclonic jerks and respiratory arrythmias are also described. Some authorities differentiate this second group of symptoms from tardive dyskinesia, preferring to categorise them as 'drug-related encephalopathies'.

Tardive dyskinesia, mainly of the BLM type, has been reported in 10 to 30 per cent of patients suffering from chronic schizophrenia. It is generally believed to be associated with long-term treatment with antipsychotic drugs and is very rarely seen before such treatment has been continuously administered for at least 6 months, and is uncommon before 4 or 5 years. While the syndrome is certainly commoner in patients on long-term antipsychotic drug treatment, it is by no means confined to them, and there are a number of well-documented patients who have never taken or been given any antipsychotic drug and yet who show unequivocal tardive dyskinesia.

Although generally suspected as being a consequence of prolonged antipsychotic drug treatment, stopping treatment may well lead to a sharp exacerbation of the symptoms; and in some patients they are observed for the first time on stopping antipsychotic drugs. This is thought to reflect an underlying increase in sensitivity of DA receptors; stopping the blockade of these supersensitive DA receptors by stopping the drug only further increases the action of DA, giving rise to the abnormal movements. It has been suggested that such a response to continuous DA receptor blockade resembles denervation super-sensitivity. It would appear that such supersensitivity is confined largely to the DA receptors in the neostriatum, for no rebound increase in psychotic symptoms is observed on stopping anti-psychotic drug treatment, nor has any fall in plasma prolactin level been detected. Furthermore, challenge of the pituitary DA receptors with haloperidol produces a rise in plasma level no different from that seen in drug-free patients. This would argue against a generalised DA receptor supersensitivity.

In view of the fact that the syndrome can be observed in patients who have never received antipsychotic drugs, and the repeated observation that it is much commoner in elderly patients, the suggestion has been made that antipsychotic drugs merely accelerate a naturally occurring degenerative process within the extrapyramidal system leading to DA receptor sensitivity. In other words, it occurs as the result of both morphological and pharmacological denervation; and it is perhaps because of the morphological element that it often persists for years after all antipsychotic drugs have been stopped.

Management of tardive dyskinesia   As tardive dyskinesia is believed to be at least partially related to an increase in the sensitivity of post-synaptic DA receptors in the corpus striatum, one possible approach would be to reduce the amount of available DA which could be released from the pre-synaptic neurones. Tetrabenazine, a compound similar in its pharmacological action to reserpine, in that it leads to depletion of the amount of catecholamines stored in the pre-synaptic vesicles, has shown some superiority over placebo when given 25 mg three to four times daily. Along the same lines, it has been suggested that, when tardive dyskinesia occurs after stopping medication with antipsychotic drugs, then resumption of antipsychotic drug treatment is indicated. We do not advocate this because, if the condition is itself a consequence of prolonged treatment with antipsychotic drugs, giving more of the same is hardly likely to improve matters in the long run, whatever the short-term gains.

As DA pathways act in the corpus striatum by inhibiting acetylcholine neurones, another strategy which has been adopted to overcome the presumed supersensitivity of the DA receptors in the dendrites of these neurones is to counter the effects of such inhibition either by increasing the synthesis or delaying the catabolism of acetyl choline. And, indeed, choline precursors such as lecithin have been shown to have some potential beneficial effect. Another putative choline precursor, deanol, was without effect, but it was subsequently shown that this drug has no effect at all on central cholinergic transmission, whereas lecithin does. Cholinesterase inhibitors, such as physostigmine, which reduce the enzymatic degradation of acetyl choline have also been shown to be of some benefit; unfortunately physostigmine has to be given by systemic injection at frequent intervals, and thus is unsuitable for continuous treatment.

Yet another possible tactic is to potentiate neurotransmission within the GABA tract leading from the corpus striatum back to the substantia nigra. Unfortunately the drugs thus far given for this purpose, such as baclofen, a direct GABA receptor agonist, and sodium valproate (Epilim), a potentiator of GABA-inergic neurotransmission, have proved to be inconsistent.

In general the most effective approach in the management of tardive dyskinesia is to stop treatment completely with antipsychotic drugs if at all possible.

As has already been stated, the symptoms may take a considerable time to remit, even up to three or four years after stopping antipsychotic drugs, and in a disturbing number of patients they appear to be permanent. Thus prevention is all-important. To this end antipsychotic drugs should be prescribed only when absolutely necessary, and then they should be administered at as low a dose and for as short a time as is consistent with amelioration of psychotic symptoms. They should be stopped, at least for a while, at the first intimation of tardive dyskinesia. An intermittent medication regime with regular so-called 'drug holidays' may be of prophylactic value although these drug holidays should not be longer than three or four weeks, otherwise relapse of schizophrenic symptoms is likely to occur.

3 Autonomic effects

(a) *Antiadrenergic* Most phenothiazines have a marked anti-adrenergic activity. This is particularly true for those with a piperidine side chain such as thioridazine. These can produce severe postural hypotension leading to circulatory collapse. Raising the foot of the bed is usually sufficient to restore cerebral

129

circulation. In extreme cases noradrenaline (*not adrenaline*) should be given by intravenous infusion.

Other cardiovascular complications of phenothiazine medication include ECG changes and frank dysrhythmias which may go on to ventricular fibrillation. These are considered to be related to a quinidine-like action of the phenothiazines, particularly thioridazine.

Of less clinical importance, but causing extreme annoyance to patients when it does occur, is failure of ejaculation. This is also more commonly a consequence of thioridazine medication than of other phenothiazines. However, this effect may be put to good use in the treatment of patients presenting with premature ejaculation (see chapter 8).

(b) *Anticholinergic* As a result of the anticholinergic action of the phenothiazines, dryness of the mouth, constipation, difficulty in micturition and blurred vision can occur.

4 Neuroleptic malignant syndrome

This is a relatively rare, but potentially fatal, idiosyncratic reaction to treatment with antipsychotic drugs. The clinical features include muscular rigidity, hyperthermia and autonomic instability. There may be associated involuntary movements, catatonic posturing and a fluctuating level of consciousness. It usually comes on within a short time after the start of treatment with antipsychotic drugs, and is more common in younger patients. The syndrome has been reported after exposure to a wide range of dopamine receptor blocking or dopamine depleting drugs given for a variety of clinical conditions; concurrent administration of lithium has been implicated in a number of cases.

It is uncertain whether the condition is central or peripheral in origin. Although muscle relaxants alone can lead to improvement, some cases require a centrally acting dopamine agonist for complete resolution, suggesting that the brain is the site where the primary abnormality occurs.

Diagnosis is based entirely on clinical grounds, CSF examination and brain CT scans are normal, the EEG may reveal non-specific slow waves, and plasma creatinine phosphokinase may be elevated as a consequence of muscle necrosis.

Immediately neuroleptic malignant syndrome is suspected, all antipsychotic drugs must be stopped. Active steps should be taken to reduce body temperature by cooling and dehydration corrected. Combined administration of the muscle relaxant drug dantrolene (10 mg/kg) and the centrally acting dopamine receptor agonist bromocriptine (up to 60 mg daily) is the treatment of choice.

5   Metabolic effects

(a)   *Weight gain*   There is often considerable weight gain noted by patients on phenothiazines, particularly chlorpromazine. The pathogenesis of this is not known, but many patients report a marked increase in hunger, and this, together with the reduction in activity caused by the sedative effect of the drug, may well account for the gain in weight.

Weight gain, often amounting to frank obesity is disturbingly common among patients receiving long-term depot antipsychotics. In one survey over a third were categorised as being clinically obese on the basis of their Body Mass Index (weight (kg) ÷ height^2 (m)). There is some suggestion that haloperidol decanoate is less likely to cause weight gain. Among the longer-acting oral preparations pimozide is less prone to promote an increase in body weight. This may be because of its relatively specific pharmacological profile; unlike phenothiazine compounds it does not block 5–HT receptors.

When weight gain becomes troublesome a low-calorie diet should be instituted. The non-stimulant appetite suppressant, fenfluramine (Ponderax) (see chapter 12), has been shown to be of benefit in helping such patients lose weight.

(b)   *Endocrine*   Antipsychotic drugs have been implicated as a cause of menstrual irregularity, and of lactation in non-pregnant women. Reduced libido or impotence can occur in the male. This is presumably secondary to drug-induced hyperprolactinaemia.

(c)   *Pigmentation*   Possibly as a result of the catalytic effect of ultraviolent light acting upon the melanin in the skin in the presence of phenothiazines, melanin may be deposited in the exposed skin. This leads to the purplish pigmentation in these areas which may be seen in patients receiving high doses of chlorpromazine for long periods. Melanin deposits may also be found in the cornea and in the lens of the eye. D-penicillamine in a dose of 1 g daily is said to be effective in reducing this pigmentation. In addition, thioridazine in high dosage can produce pigmentary retinopathy.

6 Convulsant activity

The epileptic seizure threshold is reduced by administration of phenothiazine drugs, and fits may occur even in patients without a previous epileptic history, while known epileptics show an increase in fit frequency.

7 Hypersensitivity reactions

(a) *Cholestatic jaundice* Some patients receiving chlorpromazine develop jaundice of the cholestatic type within a few weeks of starting medication. The incidence of the complication, at one time reported to be about 1 per cent of all patients given chlorpromazine, appears to have fallen considerably in recent years. When chlorpromazine-induced jaundice does occur the drug must be stopped immediately. The jaundice then nearly always subsides spontaneously within a few weeks. If necessary, another neuro-leptic drug may be given when liver function has returned to normal.

(b) *Leukopenia* A fall in the total white cell count which may progress to fatal agranulocytosis occurs in a tiny minority of patients on phenothiazines (perhaps one to four in every million patients). Unfortunately, when it does happen the onset is rapid; routine monitoring of the total white cell count is therefore unlikely to pick it up in time. Any patient on phenothiazines (particularly chlorpromazine) complaining of a sore throat or fever, should have an immediate haematological investigation. If a fall in the leucocyte count is found, the drug must be stopped straight away and a full course of antibiotic treatment begun. Even with energetic treatment the mortality rate may be as high as 50 per cent. If the patient survives, extreme caution should be taken before prescribing any neuroleptic drug again.

(c) *Skin reactions* Urticarial sensitivity rashes are not uncommon after neuroleptic medication. In addition, light-sensitive dermatoses may lead to an erythematous response of the exposed skin, or a

more serious eczematous rash. Protecting the skin from sunlight is
the only sure way of avoiding complication. Barrier creams are of
limited value.

Table 8 *Neuroleptic drugs*

Approved name	Proprietary name	Recommended dose (daily unless stated otherwise)	Remarks
phenothiazines 1 *aliphatic side chain*			
chlorpromazine	Largactil, Thorazine	Acutely disturbed patient: 300–900 mg Maintenance therapy: 100–500 mg	The standard phenothiazine. As effective as all other neuroleptics in the treatment of schizophrenia. But more marked tendency to produce drowsiness and risk of cholestatic jaundice and blood dyscrasias rather higher
promazine	Sparine	150–300 mg	Least effective of the phenothiazines, and more sedative. Useful for reducing disturbed behaviour in the elderly
2 *piperidine side chain*			
thioridazine	Melleril	150–600 mg	As effective as chlorpromazine with less tendency to produce extrapyramidal symptoms. More prone, however, to antiadrenergic effects such as hypotension

133

Table 8 *contd.*

Approved name	Proprietary name	Recommended dose (daily unless stated otherwise)	Remarks
			and failure of ejaculation. Thioridazine can cause retinal pigmentation in prolonged dosage
3 *piperazine side chain*			More extrapyramidal effects than other phenothiazines
prochlor-perazine	Stemetil	25–150 mg	The piperazine analogue of chlorpromazine to which it is clinically equivalent but produces decreased rather than increased appetite
trifluo-perazine	Stelazine	10–30 mg	No advantages over other phenothiazines
perphenazine	Fentazin Trilafon	12–24 mg	No obvious advantages over other phenothiazines
fluphenazine	Moditen Prolixin	2.5–15 mg	
fluphenazine enanthate	Moditen enanthate	12.5–25 mg every 1–3 weeks	Long-acting form given by deep intramuscular injection. Very useful in out-patient maintenance therapy of chronic schizophrenia
fluphenazine decanoate	Modecate	12.5–25 mg every 2–4 weeks	
pericyazine	Neulactil	7.5–90 mg	Said to be useful in the management of character disorders

Table 8   *contd.*

Approved name	Proprietary name	Recommended dose (daily unless stated otherwise)	Remarks
metho-trimeprazine	Veractil	15–100 mg	No obvious advantage over the other phenothiazines
pipothiazine palmitate	Piportil Depot	50–100 mg every 4 weeks	Long-acting depot preparation
thioxanthenes chlor-prothixene	Taractan	50–300 mg	Thioxanthene analogue of chlorpromaine. Possibly slightly inferior to chlorpromazine in acute schizophrenia
clopenthixol	Clopixol	100–400 mg	Thioxanthene analogue of perphenazine to which it may be equal in efficacy, although also said to be inferior to chlorpromazine
clopenthixol decoanate	Clopixol concentrate	500 mg every 1–4 weeks	
thiothixene	Navane	10–30 mg	Thioxanthene analogue of thioproperazine. As effective as phenothiazines but prone to cause extrapyramidal effects
flupenthixol	Fluanxol	3–12 mg	Thioxanthene analogue of fluphenazine to which it is equal in efficacy

Table 8 *contd.*

Approved name	Proprietary name	Recommended dose (daily unless stated otherwise)	Remarks
flupenthixol decanoate	Depixol	20–40 mg every 1–3 weeks	Long-acting form of flupenthixol useful for maintenance therapy of chronic schizophrenia. Possibly less likely to cause depression than fluphenazine decanoate
indole derivatives oxypertine	Integrin	20–60 mg	Equal to phenothiazines in efficacy in schizophrenia. Effective in lower dose in treatment of anxiety
butyrophenones haloperidol	Serenace Haldol	1–12 mg	As effective as phenothiazines in schizophrenia, but very prone to cause extrapyramidal symptoms. Said to be particularly effective in mania. In low dosage may help in anxiety
haloperidol decoanate	Haldol decoanate	50–200 mg every 1–4 weeks	Long-acting form of haloperidol. Useful for maintenance therapy of chronic schizophrenia. Possibly less likely to cause weight gain than other depot medications
trifluperidol (triperidol)	Triperidol	1–3 mg	Possibly among the most effective neuroleptics, having

Table 8   *contd.*

Approved name	Proprietary name	Recommended dose (daily unless stated otherwise)	Remarks
			been shown to be superior to chlorpromazine, but not to trifluoperazine
benperidol (benzperidol)	Frenactil	2–6 mg	Less effective than chlorpromazine in schizophrenia. Appears to reduce sexual drive, and thus may be of some use in the treatment of sexual offenders
droperidol	Droleptan	5–20 mg iv (a single dose)	Rapidly acting – useful for emergency management of acutely disturbed behaviour
diphenylbutylpiperidines pimozide	Orap	4–40 mg	As effective as phenothiazines in schizophrenia. Main advantage is that it only needs to be given once daily. Also effective in maintenance treatment of chronic schizophrenia
fluspirilene	Imap Redeptin	2–6 mg weekly	Long-acting compound. Administered once weekly by intramuscular injection. Used in maintenance therapy of chronic schizophrenia

CLINICAL APPLICATIONS

Table 8 *contd.*

Approved name	~Proprietary name	Recommended dose (daily unless stated otherwise)	Remarks
benzamides sulpiride	Dolmatil	600–1800 mg	As effective as phenothiazines in schizophrenia. May be less likely to cause tardive dyskinesia

Suggestions for further reading

Schizophrenia – general

CROW, T. J., 'Molecular pathology of schizophrenia: more than the disease process?' *British Medical Journal*, vol. 1, 1980, pp. 66–8.

Neurochemistry of schizophrenia

ANGRIST, B., THOMPSON, H., SHOPSIN, B., and GERSHAW, S., 'Clinical studies with dopamine receptor stimulants', *Psychopharmacologia*, vol. 44, 1975, pp. 273–80.

CARLSSON, A., 'Does dopamine play a role in schizophrenia?' *Psychological Medicine*, vol. 7, 1977, pp. 583–97.

CROW, T. J., JOHNSTONE, E. C., and MCCLELLAND, H. A., 'The coincidence of schizophrenia and Parkinsonism: some neurochemical implications', *Psychological Medicine*, vol. 6, 1976, pp. 227–33.

OWEN, F., CRAWLEY, J., CROSS, A. J., CROW, T. J., *et al.*, 'Dopamine D_2 receptors and schizophrenia', in *Psychopharmacology: Recent Advances and Future Prospects*, ed. S. Iversen, Oxford University Press, Oxford, 1985, pp. 216–17.

POST, R. M., FINK, E., CARPENTER, W. T., and GOODWIN, F. K., 'Cerebro-spinal fluid amine metabolites in acute schizophrenia', *Archives of General Psychiatry*, vol. 32, 1975, pp. 1063–9.

Pharmacology of antipsychotic drugs

ANDÉN, N. E., BUTCHER, S. G., CORRODI, H., FUXE, F., and UNGERSTEDT, U., 'Receptor activity and turnover of dopamine and noradrenaline after neuroleptics', *European Journal of Pharmacology*, vol. 11, 1970, pp. 303–14.

138

ANTLEMAN, S. M., SZECHTMAN, H., CHIN, P., and FISHER, A. E., 'Inhibition of tyrosine hydroxylase but not dopamine-beta-hydroxylase facilitates the action of behaviourally ineffective doses of neuroleptics', *Journal of Pharmacy and Pharmacology*, vol. 28, 1976, pp. 66–8.

BUNNEY, W. E., and AGHAJANIAN, G. K., 'A comparison of the effects of chlorpromazine, 7-hydroxychlorpromazine and chlorpromazine sulfoxide on the activity of central dopaminergic neurones', *Life Science*, vol. 15, 1974, p. 309.

CARLSSON, A., 'Antipsychotic drugs and catecholamine synapses', *Journal of Psychiatric Research*, vol. 11, 1974, pp. 57–64.

CREECE, I., BURT, D. R., and SNYDER, S. H., 'Biochemical actions of neuroleptic drugs', in *Handbook of Psychopharmacology*, vol. 10, ed. L. I. Iversen, S. D. Iversen and S. H. Snyder, Plenum Press, New York, 1978, pp. 37–89.

CROW, T. J., DEAKIN, J. F. W., and LONDON, A., 'Do anti-psychotic drugs act by dopamine receptor blockade in the nucleus accumbens?', *British Journal of Pharmacology*, vol. 52, 1976, pp. 60–1.

GRAHAME-SMITH, D. G., and ORR, M. W., 'Clinical psychopharmacology', in *Recent Advances in Clinical Pharmacology*, vol. 1, ed. P. Turner and D. G. Shand, Churchill Livingstone, Edinburgh, 1978.

JENNER, P., and MARSDEN, C. D., 'The substituted benzamides – a novel class of dopamine antagonists', *Life Sciences*, vol. 25, 1979, pp. 479–86.

SCHOOLER, N. R., SAKALIS, G., CHAN, T. L., GERSHON, S., GOLDBERG, S. C., and COLLINS, P., 'Chlorpromazine metabolism and clinical response in acute schizophrenia', in *Pharmacokinetics of Psychoactive Drugs*, ed. L. A. Gottschalk and S. Merlis, Spectrum, New York, 1976, pp. 199–219.

Neuroendocrinology of antipsychotic drugs

COTES, P. M., CROW, T. J., JOHNSTONE, E. C., BARTLETT, W., and BOURNE, R. C., 'Neuroendocrine changes in acute schizophrenia as a function of clinical state and neuroleptic medication', *Psychological Medicine*, vol. 8, 1978, pp. 657–65.

KOLAKOWSKA, T., ORR, M., GELDER, M., HEGGIE, M., WILES, D., and FRANKLIN, M., 'Clinical significance of plasma drug and prolactin levels during acute chlorpromazine treatment', *British Journal of Psychiatry*, vol. 135, 1979, pp. 352–9.

RAO, V. A. R., BISHOP, M., and COLLON, A., 'Clinical state, plasma levels of haloperidol and prolactin: a correlation study in chronic schizophrenia', *British Journal of Psychiatry*, vol. 137, 1980, pp. 518–21.

Drug treatment in schizophrenia

CROW, T. J., MACMILLAN, J. F., JOHNSON, A. L., and JOHNSTONE, E. C., 'The Northwick Park Study of first episodes of schizophrenia: a randomised controlled trial of prophylactic neuroleptic treatment', *British Journal of Psychiatry*, vol. 148, 1986, pp. 120–7.

CURSON, D. A., BARNES, T. R. E., BAMBER, R. W., PLATT, S. D., HIRSCH, S. R., and DUFFY, J. C., 'Long term depot maintenance of chronic schizophrenic out-patients', *British Journal of Psychiatry*, vol. 146, 1986, pp. 464–80.

DAHL, S. G., 'Plasma level monitoring of antipsychotic drugs: clinical utility', *Clinical Pharmacokinetics*, vol. 11, 1986, pp. 36–61.

DAVIS, J. M., and GARVIER, D. L., 'Neuroleptics: clinical use in psychiatry', in *Handbook of Psychopharmacology*, vol. 10, ed. L. I. Iversen, S. D. Iversen and S. H. Snyder, Plenum Press, New York, 1978, pp. 129–64.

DAWSON, D. A. W., 'The expectation of outcome from maintenance therapy in chronic schizophrenic patients', *British Journal of Psychiatry*, vol. 128, 1976, pp. 246–50.

ECCLESTON, D., FAIRBAIRN, A. F., HASSANYEH, F., MCCLELLAND, H. A., and STEPHENS, D. A., 'The effects of propranolol and thioridazine on positive and negative symptoms of schizophrenia', *British Journal of Psychiatry*, vol. 147, 1985, pp. 623–30.

EDWARDS, J. S., ALEXANDER, J. R., ALEXANDER, M. S., GORDON, A., and ZUTCHI, T., 'Controlled trial of sulpiride in chronic schizophrenic patients', *British Journal of Psychiatry*, vol. 137, 1980, pp. 522–9.

FALLOON, I., WATT, D. C., and SHEPHERD, M., 'A controlled trial of pimozide and fluphenazine decanoate', *Psychological Medicine*, vol. 8, 1978, pp. 59–70.

GERLACH, J., BEHULCE, K., HELTBERG, J., MUNK-ANDERSON, E., and NEILSEN, J., 'Sulpiride and Haloperidol in schizophrenia', *British Journal of Psychiatry*, vol. 147, 1985, pp. 283–88.

JOHNSON, D. A. W., 'The long-acting depot neuroleptics', in *Recent Advances in Clinical Psychiatry*, vol. 4, ed. K. Granville-Grossman, Churchill Livingstone, Edinburgh, 1982, pp. 243–60.

MACKAY, A. V. P., 'Assessment of anti-psychotic drugs', *British Journal of Clinical Pharmacology*, vol. 11, 1981, pp. 225–36.

MCINTYRE, I. M., and GERSHON, S., 'Interpatient variations in antipsychotic therapy', *Journal of Clinical Psychiatry*, vol. 46, 1985, pp. 3–5.

MCREADIE, E., MACKIE, M., MORRISON, D., and KIDD, J., 'Once weekly pimozide versus fluphenazine decanoate as maintenance therapy in chronic schizophrenia', *British Journal of Psychiatry*, vol. 140, 1982, pp. 280–6.

MANCHANDA, R., and HIRSCH, S. R., 'Does propranolol have an antipsychotic effect?' *British Journal of Psychiatry*, vol. 148, 1986, pp. 701–7.

PETRIE, W. M., and BAN, T., 'Vitamins in psychiatry: do they have a role?' *Drugs*, vol. 30, 1985, pp. 58–65.

SIMPSON, G. M., and YADALAM, K., 'Blood levels of neuroleptics: state of the art', *Journal of Clinical Psychiatry*, vol. 46, 1985, pp. 22–8.

SINGH, M., and KAY, S. R., 'A longitudinal therapeutic comparison between two prototypic neuroleptics (haloperidol and chlorpromazine) in matched groups of schizophrenics', *Psychopharmacologia*, vol. 43, 1975, pp. 115–23.

SWAZEY, J. P., *Chlorpromazine in Psychiatry*, MIT Press, Cambridge, Mass., 1974.

WISTEDT, B., 'A comparative trial of haloperidol decanoate and fluphenazine decoanate in chronic schizophrenic patients', *International Clinical Psychopharmacology*, vol. 1, supplement 1, 1986, pp. 15–23.

WISTEDT, B., and RANTA, J., 'Comparative double-blind study of flupenthixol decanoate and fluphenazine decanoate in the treatment of patients relapsing in a schizophrenic symptomatology', *Acta Psychiatrica Scandinavica*, vol. 67, 1983, pp. 378–8.

Unwanted effects of antipsychotic drugs

ABBOTT, R. J., and LOIZOU, L. A., 'Neuroleptic Malignant Syndrome', *British Journal of Psychiatry*, vol. 148, 1986, pp. 47–51.

ADLER, L., ANGRIST, B., PESELOW, E., CORWIN, J., MASLANSKY, R., and ROTROSEN, J., 'A controlled assessment of propranolol in the treatment of neuroleptic-induced akathisia', *British Journal of Psychiatry*, vol. 149, 1986, pp. 42–5.

BARNES, T. R. E., and BRAUDE, W. M., 'Akathisia variants and tardive dyskinesia', *Archives of General Psychiatry*, vol. 42, 1985, pp. 874–8.

BRAUDE, W. M., BARNES, T. R. E., and GORE, S. M., 'Clinical characteristics of akathisia', *British Journal of Psychiatry*, vol. 143, 1983, pp. 139–50.

CASEY, D. E., CHASE, T. N., CHRISTENSEN, A. V., and GERLACH, J., *Dyskinesia: research and treatment*, Springer-Verlag, Berlin, 1985.

CRAWSHAW, J. A., and MULLEN, P. E., 'A study of benzhexol abuse', *British Journal of Psychiatry*, vol. 145, 1984, pp. 300–3.

KANE, J. M., and SMITH, J.M., 'Tardive dyskinesia', *Archives of General Psychiatry*, vol. 39, 1982, pp. 473–81.

LANCET, EDITORIAL, 'Neuroleptic Malignant Syndrome', *Lancet*, vol. 1, 1984, pp. 545–6.

LITVAK, R., and KAELBLING, R., 'Agranulocytosis, leukopenia and psychotropic drugs', *Archives of General Psychiatry*, vol. 24, 1971, pp. 265–7.

MACKAY, A. V. P., and SHEPPARD, G. P., 'Pharmacotherapeutic trials in tardive dyskinesia', *British Journal of Psychiatry*, vol. 135, 1979, pp. 489–99.

MARSDEN, C. D., and JENNER, P., 'The pathophysiology of extrapyramidal side-effects of neuroleptic drugs', *Psychological Medicine*, vol. 10, 1980, pp. 55–72.

MARSDEN, C. D., and SCHACHTER, M., 'Assessment of extrapyramidal disorders', *British Journal of Clinical Pharmacology*, vol. 11, 1981, pp. 129–51.

POLLEN, G. P., BEST, N. R., and MAGUIRE, J., 'Anticholinergic drug abuse; a common problem?' *British Medical Journal*, vol. X, 1984, pp. 612–13.

SILVERSTONE, T., 'Psychotropic drugs, appetite and body weight', in *Psychopharmacology and Food*, eds M. Sander and T. Silverstone, Oxford University Press, Oxford, 1985, pp. 139–45.

Affective disorders

7

And men should know that from the brain comes joys, delights, laughter and jests, and sorrows, griefs, despondency and lamentations.

Hippocrates

Introduction

The affective disorders are those conditions in which there is alteration of mood to such a degree as to cause serious distress or disruption of normal life. The mood may be abnormally elevated as in mania, or lowered as in depression. Depression may either be a symptom of reaction to adverse circumstances, or an illness in its own right. The tendency to confuse the symptom with the illness has in the past led to certain conceptual difficulties. We all get depressed (symptom) from time to time when things go wrong; this is a perfectly natural reaction. Some people react rather more frequently and sharply than others, but the quality of their *depressive reaction* does not differ from our own. A few people, however, (1–2 per cent of the population) develop a much more serious condition – a true *depressive illness* which, as often as not, comes completely out of the blue with no obvious precipitating cause. A number of labels have been given to this illness: 'melancholia', 'psychotic depression', 'the depressive phase of a maniac–depressive psychosis', 'endogenous depression', and, when it comes on later in life, 'involutional melancholia'. Essentially, however, they are all similar in their manifestation and the basic treatment approach is the same for each. Only when states of depression alternate with episodes of mania should the term 'manic–depressive psychosis' be used. Some authors refer to the depressive phase of this particular variant as 'bipolar' depression, reserving 'unipolar' depression for those cases in which mania has not previously appeared.

The American Psychiatric Association's *Diagnostic and Statistical Manual* (*DSM III*) categorises depressive illness as a 'major depressive episode' which in its more severe forms is labelled as 'with melancholia'.

Psychopathology

Depressive illness (DSM III – *major depressive episode*)

This can be described as a persistent alteration of mood, exceeding customary sadness, which characteristically comes on 'out of the blue' with no obvious environmental precipitant. It is usually accompanied by one or more of the following symptoms: self-deprecation and a morbid sense (or delusional ideas) of guilt; sleep disturbance (typically early morning awakening); retardation of thought or action; agitated behaviour; suicidal ideas or attempts at suicide; an inability to concentrate and lack of interest in the surroundings; profound anorexia with consequent weight loss. It does not change with alteration in environmental circumstance and requires treatment with drugs or electroconvulsive therapy (ECT).

Depressive reaction

This, on the other hand, can clearly be seen to arise as the direct result of some unfortunate circumstance in the patient's life. Typically the patient blames others for his misfortune rather than himself. (In contrast, the patient with depressive illness is usually riddled with self-blame.) In a depressive reaction there are no delusional ideas, severe retardation is uncommon and successful suicide occurs far less frequently. The sleep disturbance is characteristically a difficulty in getting off to sleep rather than early morning waking. Although anorexia may occur in some patients, others turn to food for comfort and thus gain, rather than lose, weight. Finally, depressive reactions readily respond to environmental changes, and if the precipitating circumstances can be alleviated further treatment often proves unnecessary.

Mania (DSM III – *manic episode*)

Mania occurs less frequently than depression. It is characterised by overactivity both day and night, loss of social inhibitions and lack of judgment leading to self-assertiveness, over-generosity and recklessness. In addition, the manic patient has a sense of well-being and talks non-stop in a continuous stream of jokes, puns and personal remarks, which very soon become extremely wearisome to the listener. While some cases abort spontaneously, most require medical intervention.

Biochemical basis of affective disorders

Both depressive illness and mania are associated with biochemical changes in the brain and other parts of the body which are of importance in pathogenesis and in further development of the disorder. These changes involve particularly the brain amines, the electrolytes sodium and potassium, and certain hormones, particularly thyroid and adrenocorticosteroid hormones.

Monoamines

Following the largely unexpected observations that imipramine, a drug originally synthesised as a neuroleptic, had pronounced antidepressant activity, and that iproniazid, a drug used in the treatment of tuberculosis, had euphoriant properties (see chapter 1), a determined effort was made to understand how these drugs acted in the brain, in the hope of discovering the neurochemical basis of the affective disorders. It was a case of empirical treatments in search of rational explanations.

Imipramine was found to inhibit the neuronal reuptake of noradrenaline (NA) and 5–hydroxytryptamine (5–HT) by pre-synaptic neurones in the CNS (see chapter 2). Iproniazid was shown to inhibit the enzyme monoamine oxidase within the neurone; this enzyme is responsible for metabolising all three neurotransmitter monoamines. Subsequently this and other compounds with similar inhibitory activity on monoamine oxidase came to be known as monoamine oxidase inhibitors (MAOI).

At about the same time, reserpine, a compound which had been introduced in the early 1950s for the treatment of hypertension, was noted to cause symptoms resembling a severe depressive illness in a number of patients. Examination of its action in the CNS revealed that reserpine depleted the brain stores of the three monoamine neurotransmitters, NA, dopamine (DA) and 5–HT. Thus, a drug which depleted the brain of monoamines caused

145

depression, while drugs which increased the available monoamine neurotransmitters at the receptor, either by blocking their reuptake (the dibenzazepines) or by preventing their metabolism (the MAOI), elevated mood. These observations gave rise to what has come to be known as the monoamine theory of depression, which may be stated as follows:

> Depression is due to an absolute or relative *decrease* in monoamines, or of receptor sensitivity, at certain receptor sites in the brain, whereas mania is due to an absolute or relative *excess* of monoamines, or an increase in receptor sensitivity, at these sites.

Stated in such general terms this theory still has some validity. Unfortunately it offers no clues as to which receptor sites or which monoamines are involved. In any case depression is unlikely to be a unitary condition. Genetically, bipolar depression can be distinguished from unipolar, and this genetic distinction is paralleled by biochemical differences between the two types of depression. For example, levodopa, the precursor of dopamine, can produce symptoms of mania in patients with bipolar depression but not in those with unipolar depressive illness. This would suggest that DA is involved in bipolar, but not in unipolar depression. In other words bipolar depression may be associated with a decrease in DA activity, and mania might be associated with an increase. The finding that pimozide, a specific dopamine receptor blocking compound, is effective in mania is consistent with such a view. Unipolar depression on the other hand may be due to a reduction in the activity of either an NA system, or a 5–HT system, or both.

5–HT was first implicated in the pathogenesis of depression by the finding of a lowered level of 5–hydroxyindoleacetic acid (5–HIAA) (the metabolite of 5–HT) in the CSF in some depressed patients and the reduction in the concentration of 5–HT in the brains of suicides. It now appears that these changes relate more to suicidal behaviour and impulsivity than to depression itself. However 5–HT is still thought to be concerned in depressive illness, with some of the antidepressant drugs acting at least partly by increasing central 5–HT neurotransmission (see below).

Noradrenaline has been imputed to be involved in the pathogenesis of depressive illness by a number of authorities. This view is based on the finding that the urinary concentration of the metabolites of NA, 3 methoxy, -4-hydroxy-phenylglycol (MHPG) and vanilylmandelic acid (VMA) was reduced in depressed patients. Subsequent investigations suggested that the reduction in these metabolites of NA was secondary to the generalised reduction in overall motor activity which occurs in retarded depressed patients. In any case there is no firm evidence that even the CSF MHPG level is a true reflection of NA activity in the brain; it may be more closely related to spinal cord activity. A reduction in the uptake of 5–HT and dopamine by platelets of patients with depression, together with increased sensitivity to the pressor effects of intravenous tyramine, when compared with matched control subjects, has been described, but the biochemical basis for these changes in monoamine activity is not known. Similarly, the clinical significance of decreased platelet MAO activity in depression is uncertain. Yet, in spite of these doubts concerning the role of NA in depression it should be stated that the drugs which appear to act most rapidly in depressive illness, drugs such as protriptyline and maprotiline, are believed to act largely if not entirely on the NA system. Furthermore amphetamine, which can alleviate depressive symptoms in a number of patients, albeit for a short time, acts almost exclusively on the catecholamines NA and DA. It may well be that unipolar depressive illness can arise as a consequence of a number of biochemical abnormalities; in some patients it may well be due to changes in the 5–HT system, in others the NA system may be affected, while in yet others altogether different neuro-transmitter systems might play a part.

In any case 5–HT appears to facilitate NA neurotransmission, and presumably the converse is true, that a reduction in 5–HT leads to a lowering of NA neurotransmission. There is endocrino-logical evidence that the reactivity of at least some central NA pathways is reduced (see below). One suggestion is that this comes about as a result of an increased sensitivity of pre-synaptic alpha-2 receptors, thereby lowering the synthesis of NA (see chapter 2).

Cholinergic mechanism

The possible involvement of disturbances in cholinergic trans-mission should not be overlooked. Blockade of central choline esterase with physostigmine can produce lethargy and dysphoria in normal subjects; similar treatment in patients with mania ameliorates their symptoms. Many antidepressive drugs of the monoamine reuptake inhibiting group possess strong anticholinergic properties that might be thought to contribute to their therapeutic activity, but if the group as a whole is considered, antidepressive activity does not appear to be related to anticholinergic activity.

Electrolytes

In 1932 Gjessing showed that changes in water and electrolyte balance accompanied cyclic affective disorders in some patients. Further studies, however, have produced conflicting results, because although marked changes were demonstrated, no consistent pattern has been demonstrated in particular mental states in different patients.

Endocrine function

While profound psychological changes may accompany all endocrine disorders, thyroid and adrenal cortical dysfunction in particular are associated with changes in mood. It is possible that thyroid hormone influences central nervous activity through changes in adenylcyclase, an enzyme identical to, or closely related to, the adrenergic receptor. Thyroid hormone stimulates adenylcyclase, which in turn leads to an increase in cyclic AMP. It is reasonable to suppose that changes in concentration of adenylcyclase and cyclic AMP in the brain may underlie some if not all of the psychological changes associated with a deficiency or excess of thyroid hormone. In depressive illness a frequent finding is a reduction in the response of the pituitary to the administration of thyrotrophin release hormone (TRH); less thyroid stimulating hormone (TSH) is released from the pituitary into the circulation, as determined by plasma TSH levels, in response to the intravenous injection of 0.4 mg TRH. This abnormality of the TRH test is seen in approximately 25 per cent of severely depressed patients; while in some it is probably secondary to the elevated levels of plasma cortisol seen in this condition (see below), in others this explanation does not appear to apply.

A relationship between depression and adrenal cortical activity is suggested first by the clinical observation that states of profound depression may be produced by administration of high doses of corticotrophin or cortisol. Second, patients with severe endogenous depression may themselves frequently have raised plasma cortisol levels throughout the 24 hours, with a loss of normal diurnal variation. This is probably due, in turn, to an increased pituitary corticotrophin production which may depend on disordered hypothalamic control of anterior pituitary function. Consistent with this view is the finding that the elevation in the plasma cortisol levels seen in approximately 50 per cent of severely depressed patients is, in a proportion of them, resistant to suppression by dexamethasone, a synthetic analogue of cortisol. Dexamethasone, when administered intramuscularly at a dose of 1 or 2 mg at 23.00 hours normally suppresses ACTH production through a central feed-back mechanism and as a result cortisol excretion over the subsequent 24 hours is reduced. In about 25 per cent of patients suffering from depressive illness (endogenous depression) dexamethasone fails to suppress plasma cortisol levels, presumably because of an underlying increase in the output of cortisol releasing factor (CRF) from the hypothalamus. This lack of suppression is much less frequently observed in depressive reactions (i.e. non-endogenous depression) and the dexamethasone suppression test is regarded by some authors as being a reliable discriminator between the two types of depression. However, plasma cortisol levels are also elevated in severe mania, suggesting that it is more likely to reflect a non-specific neuroendocrine response to major alterations of mood, than to be linked specifically to depressive illness.

Dexamphetamine, a drug which promotes the release of both NA and DA from pre-synaptic neurones, in normal subjects leads to an elevation of plasma cortisol. It is believed that this effect is mediated by NA pathways as it is inhibited by the NA receptor-blocking drug thymoxamine. The finding that in depressed patients dexamphetamine does not elevate plasma cortisol suggests that there might be an underlying abnormality in at least some central noradrenergic neurotransmitter systems. The finding of a reduced growth hormone response to the noradrenergic alpha-2 receptor agonist clonidine in depression also points to the involvement of NA pathways. This reduced cortisol response to dexamphetamine returns to normal on recovery. Looking at it the other way round, patients with Cushing's syndrome, whose primary abnormality is a raised level of circulating corticosteroids, frequently become profoundly depressed; this depression is improved dramatically when their endocrine state is returned to normal.

149

5–HT related endocrine responses can also be affected in depressive illness. The administration of the 5–HT precursor tryptophan causes a rise in the level of circulating prolactin in normal subjects. This response is blunted in depressed patients, although the deviation from normal is less in patients who have lost a significant amount of weight.

It is clear from the foregoing observations that a close relationship exists between mood, endocrine function and central neurotransmitter pathways. Although many of the neurotransmitter substances and neuropeptides implicated in depression can directly or indirectly influence the activity of the hypothalamus in producing releasing or inhibiting factors, which in turn affect the release of hormones from the pituitary, the exact relevance of these extremely complex interactions to the pathogenesis and response to treatment of the primary affective disorders remains uncertain.

Pharmacology

Drugs for depression

It follows from the monoamine theory of depression that successful treatment of depression should be associated with an increase in central monoamine activity or in changed monoaminergic receptor number of sensitivity. This could theoretically be achieved by several different pharmacological mechanisms (see chapter 2): (1) administration of monoamine precursors, (2) monoamine reuptake inhibition, (3) monoamine oxidase inhibition, (4) monoamine release, (5) pre-synaptic receptor blockade, (6) post-synaptic receptor stimulation, (7) phosphodiesterase inhibition.

1 *Administration of monoamine precursors* Oral or parenteral administration of the monoamine neurotransmitters is ineffective because they do not pass the blood–brain barrier, and, in any case, have powerful peripheral effects. An appropriate precursor, however, might be expected to reach the brain and increase transmitter synthesis. In the case of 5–HT, this would be either L-5-hydroxytryptophan or L-tryptophan, and it is the latter that has received most attention. The evidence from a large number of clinical trials is conflicting both for L-tryptophan alone, or in combination with lithium or MAO inhibitors. Striking results have been reported in individual patients, but overall the results have

been disappointing and it must be considered, at best, a weak antidepressive agent.

L-dopa is a precursor of dopamine and noradrenaline, and is used in treatment of Parkinson's disease. Although it can improve mood in parkinsonian patients, its usefulness in other patients has not been confirmed. Furthermore, its central biochemical effects are complex, for in addition to increasing brain dopamine content it affects 5–HT neurones and turnover.

2   *Monoamine reuptake inhibiting drugs (MARI)*   This category of drugs includes those compounds which are commonly known as the 'tricyclic antidepressants'. They have many pharmacological properties including anticholinergic, anti-5–HT, antihistamine, hypothermic and antiemetic actions. Their antidepressant activity, however, is probably largely due to their ability to block the neuronal uptake of catecholamines and 5–HT thus increasing the effective concentrations of these monoamines at central receptor sites, even though the brain amine content is not increased. It is probable that these compounds have both an acute action and a longer-term chronic effect. After a single dose they inhibit the uptake of noradrenaline and/or 5–HT in the animal brain and may also prevent deamination by monoamine oxidase in the mito-chondria. They also inhibit the pressor response to tyramine in man, and the uptake of dopamine into human platelets after administration of single doses. After administration of MARI to experimental animals for several days the uptake of monoamines is still reduced, and the levels of their metabolites are also reduced (as after acute administration). In contrast to the acute experi-ments, however, their rate of disappearance is *not* reduced, suggesting increased turnover. Furthermore, chronic administra-tion of MARI as well as of monoamine oxidase inhibitors, and of ECT to experimental animals results in a reduction in activity of the noradrenergic cyclic AMP generating system in the limbic forebrain. It may be that it is these delayed changes in monoamine turnover and in receptor activity which underlie the therapeutic activity of MARI in man, which does not usually come on until several days after administration.

Many MARI also potentiate the peripheral pressor effect of noradrenaline and adrenaline, as well as affecting their central actions. This peripheral action assumes particular importance in patients given injections of local anaesthetic preparations which contain these catecholamines, and other directly acting sympatho-mimetic pressor amines, as vaso-constrictor agents. Another important peripheral interaction of MARI is with antihypertensive drugs such as guanethidine, bethanidine and debrisoquine which block noradrenaline release after being taken up into the noradrenergic neurone. The uptake of these drugs, like that of noradrenaline, is blocked by MARI, and so their antihypertensive effect is reduced or abolished.

Many MARI possess potent anticholinergic activity, which may be related to their clinical effect, particularly if, as has been suggested, there is a disturbance of central cholinergic activity in depressive illness. Such anticholinergic activity may also underlie the cardiotoxic effect of some of these drugs.

There is increasing evidence that histamine is an important neurotransmitter in the brain (page 15) and many antidepressants of the MARI type are potent histamine antagonists. However, some drugs with marked central antihistamine activity do not possess antidepressant activity and it is unlikely to be a dominant mechanism of therapeutic action of antidepressant drugs.

Imipramine is the parent compound of the group, and is meta-bolised within the body to its desmethyl derivative desipramine. Many related compounds have now been introduced, and it is claimed, largely on the basis of animal studies, that some possess selectivity of action in blocking the uptake of one monoamine rather than another; secondary amines (e.g. desipramine, pro-triptyline) appear to be more potent than tertiary amines (e.g. imipramine, amitriptyline) in blocking NA uptake whereas the tertiary amines are generally more potent in blocking 5–HT uptake. It should, however, be remembered that the tertiary amines are metabolised to secondary amines which act preferentially on inhibiting NA uptake. Furthermore, 5–HT may well itself facilitate NA release. There is some evidence that drugs such as clomipramine, with a preferential action on 5–HT neurotrans-mission, are more effective in patients who have a low level of 5–HIAA in their CSF; conversely drugs such as nortriptyline with a preferential action on NA pathways are more effective in those patients with low CSF MHPG.

Extensive metabolism to compounds with different uptake-blocking profiles may occur in man through routes different from those in animals. This consideration obviously throws considerable doubt on conclusions relating to clinical action in patients reached from *in vitro* studies in animal tissue with the parent compound alone. And in man there is considerable genetic variability with regard to metabolism, and hence to the plasma level reached after a given dose (see chapter 3). Whether or not such variation in plasma levels is related to clinical efficacy is uncertain; some authors have described a linear relationship between plasma level and clinical response, others have described an inverted 'U' shaped relationship in which higher doses appear to be less effective, and finally yet other authors have found no relationship at all between plasma levels and therapeutic effect.

The term 'tricyclic' which was applied to these drugs was always inappropriate, because other groups of centrally acting compounds such as the phenothiazines also possess a tricyclic nucleus (page 100). However, the term has become even more inappropriate with the introduction of tetracyclic antidepressive compounds such as maprotiline, and bicyclic compounds such as viloxazine, the majority of which share with the tricyclic compounds the basic pharmacological property of central monoamine reuptake inhibition. There is a wide spectrum of peripheral pharmacological activity among these drugs, ranging from a relative lack of anticholinergic and peripheral noradrenaline reuptake blocking effects with drugs such as viloxazine to the profound anticholinergic and peripheral reuptake blocking properties of amitriptyline.

Many of the original MARI antidepressant drugs, such as amitriptyline and imipramine, adversely affect the cardiovascular system; they can cause changes in blood pressure (particularly postural hypotension), produce dysrhythmias, and influence the inotropic state of the heart. Such cardiovascular effects are thought to be related to the action these drugs have on the reuptake of biogenic amines (particularly NA) within the heart, plus, in some cases, their anticholinergic, local anaesthetic or alpha-2-receptor blocking properties. The pre-synaptic blocking drugs mianserin and trazodone are probably equally safe in this respect (see below).

Other drugs may interfere with the metabolism of the MARI antidepressants and thus influence their clinical effects. For example, phenothiazines, such as chlorpromazine (see chapter 6) may block their hydroxylation, thereby increasing their plasma levels and potentiating their therapeutic activity and their side effects.

Although the principal type of monoamine reuptake is into monoaminergic neurones (Uptake$_1$) a second form of uptake also occurs by diffusion into other, non-neuronal tissues (Uptake$_2$). There is some evidence to suggest that corticosteroids may inhibit the uptake$_2$ process, and if this occurs in the central nervous system, then it may account, at least in part, for their euphoriant and antidepressant activity in debilitated and terminally-ill patients.

3 *Monoamine oxidase inhibitors (MAOI)* Inhibition of the intra-cellular enzyme monoamine oxidase (MAO) leads to an increase of the monoamines noradrenaline, dopamine and 5–HT in the brain. Any antidepressant effect MAO inhibitors may have would fit in well with the monoamine hypothesis. Many other drugs inhibit MAO to a limited extent, including cocaine and amphetamine, but their pharmacological actions do not appear to depend on this effect. The compounds in which antidepressant effects probably depend on MAO inhibition fall into two chemical groups: (i) those which are hydrazine derivatives, particularly toxic to the liver (isocarboxazid, nialamide and phenelzine) and (ii) those related to amphetamine, the most important being tranylcypromine which appears to have intrinsic sympathomimetic activity of its own. Some of this latter group of drugs, particularly trancylcypromine are also potent inhibitors of noradrenaline uptake. It is, therefore, uncertain to what extent an increased level of noradrenaline at the receptor site produced by tranylcypromine is due to inhibition of metabolic degradation of noradrenaline on the one hand and to inhibition of uptake on the other. MAOI reduce transmission through sympathetic but not parasympathetic ganglia; this can give rise to marked postural hypotension.

Monoamine oxidase is not a single entity but a group of more specific enzymes, each of which is concerned with an individual monoamine. Most of the monoamine oxidase inhibitors in general use inhibit the whole family of enzymes and thus lead to an increase in all the monoamines. However, certain MAOI, such as clorgyline and selegiline have been claimed, on the basis of animal experiments, to inhibit preferentially the enzyme responsible for one monoamine rather than another (see page 35). Both clorgyline, a selective MAO-A inhibitor, and selegiline (deprenyl), a selective MAO-B inhibitor, have been shown to possess antidepressive activity under double-blind conditions. However, both drugs appear to lose their selectivity at higher doses and there is no clear evidence that their MAO inhibitory actions were selective at the doses used in these studies.

MAO is important in the handling of many drugs and foodstuffs within the body. For this reason, drugs which inhibit the enzyme complex may have important interactions with it.

(a) *Sympathomimetic amines* After MAO inhibition, the indirectly acting amines may evoke enhanced effects both peripherally and centrally. Many easily available proprietary remedies for upper respiratory tract infections contain such amines, and thus patients taking MAO inhibitors must be cautious in their use.

(b) *Certain foodstuffs* Foods which contain pressor amines such as dopa and tyramine may produce hypertensive reactions in patients receiving MAO inhibitors. These include broad beans, which contain dopa, and certain cheeses containing large quantities of tyramine. Under normal circumstances most tyramine ingested by mouth is metabolised immediately by MAO in the intestinal mucosa and liver. Following MAO inhibition, the absorption of tyramine is increased markedly and it rapidly enters the circulation to cause prolonged release of noradrenaline and thus evoke pressor effects. Some wines, yeast products and animal livers also contain significant amounts of tyramine.

(c) *Central nervous depressant drugs* The central effects of pethidine and other narcotic compounds are prolonged in patients receiving MAOI, and excitation, rigidity, coma, changes in blood pressure, hyperpyrexia and shock may occur. This interaction can be prevented in animals by drugs such as p-chlorophenylalanine which prevent the intracerebral accumulation of 5–HT but not by compounds which reduce noradrenaline synthesis. It appears, therefore, that an increase in brain 5–HT is necessary for this interaction to occur.

(d) *Antihypertensive drugs* Some of the antihypertensive drugs, including guanethidine and bethanidine, may release noradrenaline from peripheral sympathetic nerve endings when administered in high concentration, for example, intravenously. In the absence of MAO activity, these compounds may release increased amounts of noradrenaline on to receptor sites and produce hyperexcitation and hypertension.

(e) *Monoamine reuptake inhibiting drugs*   Antidepressant drugs, such as imipramine as described above, inhibit uptake of noradrenaline and possibly 5–HT into central nerve terminals, thus increasing their activity at receptor sites. It would be expected on theoretical grounds, therefore, that MAO inhibitors might potentiate their effects, and this has been demonstrated in animal experiments. There have also been reports of serious reactions in patients treated with a combination of these two groups of compounds.

4   *Monoamine releasing drugs*   The indirectly acting sympatho-mimetic amines such as amphetamine and phenmetrazine, together with some other drugs such as methylphenidate and pemoline, probably produce central stimulation by release of dopamine and noradrenaline from, and to some extent by blockade of uptake into, NA and DA neurones. In addition, amphetamine may have a direct central dopamine receptor stimulant action. Their central stimulant effect is seen in an increase of alertness and in motor and psychological activity, together with a decrease in fatigue and varying degrees of insomnia. These effects have led to the widespread abuse of amphetamine and phenmetrazine, and these two drugs are now subject to legal restrictions in many countries. Chronic use of this group of drugs in large doses may ultimately lead to alarming psychotic symptoms with paranoid features.

These drugs cannot be considered to be as therapeutically useful antidepressive drugs as are the MARI and MAOI, because their central effects lead to anxiety, restlessness and agitation rather than normality of mood. This may be because they enhance central catecholamine activity without increasing activity of 5–HT.

5   *Pre-synaptic receptor blockade*   Release of monoamines from central neurones is influenced by pre-synaptic receptors, some of which facilitate and others inhibit transmitter release (page 23). Stimulation of pre-synaptic alpha receptors inhibits noradrenaline release, and blockade of these receptors leads to increased release. Mianserin possesses little, if any, MARI and anticholinergic properties, but appears to possess pre-synaptic alpha receptor blocking activity that may lead to increased synaptic monoamine concentrations. Trazadone is thought to act in a similar manner.

6   *Beta-2 receptor agonists*   There is some clinical evidence that the beta^{-2} receptor agonist salbutamol possesses antidepressant

properties. In animals salbutamol produces an increased utilisation of brain NA and an increased synthesis of 5–HT. These findings are compatible with salbutamol having a putative antidepressant action.

7 *Phosphodiesterase inhibitors* The enzyme phosphodiesterase is responsible for inactivating cyclic AMP which is thought to be intimately involved with mediating noradrenergic and dopaminergic receptor activity (chapter 2). Drugs which inhibit phosphodiesterase would, therefore, be expected to increase cyclic AMP activity and produce effects similar to central catecholamine activity. The methylxanthines such as caffeine, theophylline and theobromine are phosphodiesterase inhibitors, and have central stimulant properties reducing fatigue and augmenting the capacity for physical exertion. Excessive administration produces insomnia, restlessness, anxiety, headache and tremor, and dependence may develop. As with the monoamine releasing drugs, they cannot be considered as therapeutically useful antidepressive drugs.

It would appear that the pharmacological evidence currently available in general supports the monoamine hypothesis of affective disorders, although the situation is much more complex than was originally thought. Certainly as far as antidepressant drugs are concerned, their mode of action is probably based on facilitation of brain NA and/or 5–HT neurotransmission.

8 *Hormones* The relationships which have been observed between neuroendocrine function and mental state in the affective disorders (see page 148) have suggested the possibility that these conditions might respond to hormone treatment.

(a) *Thyroxine, Thyrotrophin (TRH) and Thyroid Stimulating Hormone (TSH)* Initial reports suggesting that the addition of one or the other of the thyroid-related hormones increased the effectiveness of standard antidepressant drug treatment have not been confirmed in subsequent clinical testing. However, TRH does appear to produce a short-lived elevation of mood in normal euthyroid women, possibly through a neuromodulating action on central catecholaminergic systems.

(b) *Cortisone, Adrenocorticotropic Hormone (ACTH)* No benefit has been observed when extra corticosteroids or ACTH have been given to depressed patients. This is hardly surprising in view of the fact that endogenous production of these hormones is frequently elevated in depressive illness (see page 149).

(c) *Sex hormones* Although mild depressive symptoms may occur in association with the menopause, hormone replacement therapy (HRT) with oestrogens leads to improvement in mental state in only a proportion of patients. The whole question of HRT is very controversial as the possible dangers associated with endometrial hyperplasia may outweigh any potential psychological benefit.

(d) *Endorphins and enkephalins* α-endorphin, endorphin-related compounds and enkephalins have been tried as treatments for affective disorders. The results of trials to date have been unimpressive and inconsistent.

Electroconvulsive therapy (ECT) still remains the most effective form of antidepressant treatment for severe cases. If the monoamine theory is true, then it would be expected that this form of treatment should also influence central monoamine activity. Its effect on cerebral amines in man are not known, but animal studies suggest that intermittent application of ECT leads to an increase in the sensitivity of catecholamine receptors. Whether the same applies in man is uncertain; the finding that there is no change in the endocrine response to amphetamine following a therapeutically successful course of ECT in depressed patients would not be in favour of such a mechanism.

Drugs for mania

Two types of drugs are of value in the treatment of mania, the neuroleptic compounds and lithium.

1 *Neuroleptic drugs* The pharmacology of these drugs is considered in chapter 6. Suffice it to say here that their effectiveness in mania may be explained in terms of the monoamine theory by their ability to block post-synaptic catecholaminergic receptors, particularly dopamine.

2 *Lithium* Lithium is the lightest of the alkali earth elements, coming below sodium, potassium, rubidum and caesium in terms

of atomic weight. In the body it imperfectly substitutes for sodium and potassium ions and consequently it can have profound effects on a great number of metabolic processes. While substitution by lithium for potassium and sodium may underlie its more severe toxic effects such as convulsions and coma, this is not thought to be the basis for its psychotropic activity. Toxic symptoms begin to occur when the serum concentration exceeds 1.5 mM/L, so every effort, including regular serum estimations, must be made to ensure that this upper level of 1.5 mM/L is not exceeded. Especial care should be taken whenever there is a possibility of fluid or electrolyte imbalance as in the case of persistent vomiting or diarrhoea.

Within the central nervous system lithium reduces the neurotransmitter-induced activation of adenylate cyclase at certain post synaptic receptors. Normally the neurotransmitters noradrenaline and dopamine activate adenylate cyclase, and this in turn catalyses the formation of cyclic adenosine monophosphate (AMP) from adenosine triphosphate (ATP). AMP is frequently referred to as the 'second messenger' for in many cells it mediates the changes within those cells produced by circulating hormones ('first messengers'). In the CNS the catecholamine neurotransmitters are acting similarly to hormones in the periphery, that is they are behaving as first messengers, while cyclic AMP acts as the second messenger. The reduction by lithium of the formation of cyclic AMP within cells acted upon by catecholamine neurotransmitters would be in keeping in terms of the monoamine hypothesis, with the clinical observation that lithium is effective in mania (see section on treatment of mania). It would not, however, explain any antidepressant activity that lithium may possess, nor does it fully explain its well-documented prophylactic properties (see section on prophylaxis of affective disorders). The effect of lithium on adenylate cyclase is not limited to the CNS. Other organs, notably the thyroid gland and the kidney can also be affected. In the thyroid the release of thyroid hormone from the gland induced by thyroid stimulating hormone (TSH) is mediated by cyclic AMP, and can be inhibited by lithium. The subsequent impairment of thyroxine release can, in time, lead to the development of a frank hypothyroid syndrome. In the kidney the action of antidiuretic hormone (ADH) is mediated via cyclic AMP. Lithium, by reducing adenylate cyclase activity, interferes with the antidiurectic effect of ADH, and, as a result, there is an increased flow of dilute urine, or polyuria; a condition referred to as nephrogenic diabetes insipidus. It has been suggested that interference by lithium with the effects of vasopressin (ADH) may lead to increased hypo-thalamic release of vasopressin and that this may be involved in the psychotherapeutic action of lithium.

Although a number of cyclic AMP systems in other tissues have been shown in experimental animals to be affected by lithium, the clinical implications, if any, of such findings are as yet unknown.

Recent studies in patients with depression have shown that lithium increases 5–HT uptake into platelets. If platelets are a good model for central tryptaminergic neurones (page 36), the psychotropic effect of lithium could be explained on the basis of increased uptake and storage of 5–HT by synaptosomes, so reducing its synaptic concentration in the brain.

3   *Carbamazepine*   This has been shown to be of value in the treatment and prophylaxis of mania, but its mechanism is unknown.

4   *Calcium antagonists*   Preliminary results, including some double-blind studies, in a relatively few patients, have suggested that the calcium antagonist verapamil is effective in the treatment of mania. Perhaps this is not surprising in the light of the calcium antagonist properties of classical neuroleptic drugs (page 28) which are effective in treatment of mania.

Treatment

Depression

When presented with a patient who is unhappy, perhaps weeping, obviously distressed, and who gives a history of inability to cope, a sense of hopelessness perhaps with suicidal ideas, profound anorexia and marked insomnia, it is necessary to determine first of all the likely underlying cause for these symptoms, and secondly to assess their severity. Treatment varies considerably according to the type of condition present (i.e. whether it is a true depressive illness or a depressive reaction to distressing circumstances), and to its severity. If the patient is so desperate that there is a real risk of a suicide attempt, or if he is so incapacitated by his symptoms as to be unable to care for himself adequately, hospitalisation is likely to be necessary, followed by treatment with electroconvulsive therapy (ECT). Where the patient is neither suicidal nor incapacitated, it will usually be possible to treat him with the appropriate medication as an out-patient. Although in many cases it is not possible to distinguish categorically between a depressive illness and a depressive reaction, an attempt to do so should be made, as the treatment is different for each. Depressive illness usually responds well to one of the MARI antidepressant drugs. Furthermore, the more reactive type of depressive syndrome, particularly if persistent, also appears to respond better to an antidepressant drug such as amitryptyline than to a benzodiazepine. In cases of so-called 'atypical' depression, particularly if there is a lengthy history, with failure to respond to MARI antidepressants, monoamine oxidase inhibitors may prove effective.

Depressive illness (endogenous depression: major depressive episode)

1 *Standard tricyclic, monoamine reuptake inhibitor* The so-called tricyclic antidepressant drugs are believed to act by blocking the reuptake of monoamines from the synaptic cleft, hence the term monoamine reuptake blocking drugs (MARI) (see pages 151–4). There is a large number of such drugs available (see Table 9). They are all of similar efficacy; some 60–70 per cent of patients improve on them, compared to 30–40 per cent who improve on placebo and 70–80 per cent who improve on ECT. Patients who respond best are those suffering from a clear-cut depressive illness of moderate severity, with a history of less than six months' duration. MARI take some ten to fourteen days to become fully effective.

Among the factors which influence the metabolism and plasma levels of these drugs, and hence their efficacy, are genetic predisposition, other drugs being administered at the same time (particularly barbiturate and phenothiazine compounds), and pH (acidification of the urine leading to faster excretion).

The first drugs in this group to be introduced into clinical practice, imipramine (Tofranil) and amitriptyline (Elavil, Tryptizol), while effective, are prone to cause pronounced anticholinergic side effects such as dryness of the mouth, constipation, difficulty in micturition which can lead to urinary retention in men with prostatic hypertrophy, and difficulty in

161

visual accommodation. Other untoward effects include postural hypotension and excessive sweating. Amitriptyline causes weight gain, secondary to its appetite-stimulating effect. More dangerous, especially in overdose or in patients with a pre-existing heart disease, are the cardiotoxic properties which some of these drugs possess. Amitriptyline is the most likely to cause problems in this respect; it is not uncommon to find a prolongation of the Q–T interval, which can proceed to a frank dysrhythmia or ventricular tachycardia, which in cases of overdose occasionally progresses to fatal ventricular fibrillation. In the elderly, congestive cardiac failure is not uncommon. In addition to these autonomic and cardiac effects, the tricyclics are epileptogenic and may precipitate epileptic seizures in those who are otherwise predisposed. In view of all these possible side effects, tricyclic (MARI) drugs should be used most cautiously in patients with glaucoma, prostatism, chronic heart disease and epilepsy.

Other tricyclic MARI such as dothiepin (Prothiaden), the thiapin derivative of amitriptyline, and doxepin (Sinequan), its oxepin analogue, have been shown to be less prone to cause anticholinergic effects. Lofepramine (Gamanil), a more recently introduced member of this group of drugs, similarly has little anticholinergic activity. Desipramine (Pertofran), the demethylated metabolite of imipramine, is clinically similar to the parent compound. Clomipramine (Anafranil) is said to be particularly useful in the management of phobic and obsessional states (see chapter 8).

The other MARI compounds listed in Table 9 would not appear to have any distinct advantages over those already discussed. It is better to become familiar with the dosage and effects of some two or three compounds and stick to them.

Once a patient has responded well to ECT or to a tricyclic antidepressant he should be maintained on a lower dose of a MARI drug for some six months after recovery in order to minimise the risk of relapse. Some patients with previous recurrent depressive illness have been maintained symptom free for at least two years on continuous treatment with MARI drugs.

2   *Newer antidepressant drugs*   While some of the newer antidepressants such as maptrotiline (Ludiomil), fluvoxamine and fluoxetine are MARI (selective for 5–HT), others such as mianserin (Bolvidon) and trazadone (Desyrel, Molipaxin) are not. None of

these newer preparations appears more effective than the standard antidepressants. They do, however, have different side effect profiles. Maprotiline is particularly prone to precipitate convulsions. Fluvoxamine and fluoxetine are selective blockers of 5–HT reuptake with little or no anticholinergic action or cardiotoxic properties. Both, however, can cause gastrointestinal symptoms such as nausea; this probably reflects their action on 5–HT in the gut wall. Headache is another commonly reported side effect. In contrast to amitriptyline, weight gain does not occur, in fact fluoxetine has been found to be an effective appetite suppressant for use in the management of obesity (see chapter 12). Mianserin has some distinct advantages over the standard MARI antidepressive drugs such as imipramine and amitriptyline. It possesses few, if any, anticholinergic effects and is therefore less likely to precipitate glaucoma or urinary retention in patients at risk. It appears to be less cardiotoxic than certain MARI drugs, and, as it does not interfere with monoamine uptake, it does not antagonise the antihypertensive effects of adrenergic neurone blocking drugs (such as guanethidine or bethanidine) nor potentiate the pressor effects of directly acting sympathomimetic amines such as noradrenaline and phenylephrine. Its principal adverse effect is sedation, but this can be turned to advantage to some extent by administering a single dose at night. Unfortunately there have been a number of reports of leucopenia occurring in association with mianserin; in some cases this has gone on to fatal agranulocytosis. It is therefore essential to check the white cell count in any patient on mianserin who presents with serious infection.

Trazodone (Molipaxin) has a similar clinical profile; it too has very little anticholinergic activity and appears to have a low potential for cardiotoxicity. Both these compounds, by virtue of their relative lack of anticholinergic and cardiotoxic properties, are particularly suitable for treating depressive illness in the elderly.

3 *Monoamine oxidase inhibitors (MAOI)* Earlier trials of MAOI were largely confined to patients suffering from severe depressive illness, where these drugs were found less effective than the standard tricyclic MARI. Subsequently it has been recognised that they can be very effective in the treatment of so-called 'atypical' or 'neurotic' depression where the vegetative symptoms are frequently the obverse of those seen in the more typical depressive illness, with an increase rather than a decrease in appetite and sleep.

TREATMENT CARD

Carry this card with you at all times. Show it to any doctor who may treat you other than the doctor who prescribed this medicine, and to your dentist if you require dental treatment.

INSTRUCTIONS TO PATIENTS
Please read carefully
While taking this medicine and for 14 days after your treatment finishes you must observe the following simple instructions:-

1 Do not eat CHEESE, PICKLED HERRING OR BROAD BEAN PODS.

2 Do not eat or drink BOVRIL, OXO, MARMITE or ANY SIMILAR MEAT OR YEAST EXTRACT.

3 Eat only FRESH foods and avoid food that you suspect could be stale or 'going off'. This is especially important with meat, fish, poultry or offal. Avoid game.

4 Do not take any other MEDICINES (including tablets, capsules, nose drops, inhalations or suppositories) whether purchased by you or previously prescribed by your doctor, without first consulting your doctor or your pharmacist.
   NB *Treatment for coughs and colds, pain relievers, tonics and laxatives are medicines.*

5 Avoid alcoholic drinks.

Keep a careful note of any food or drink that disagrees with you, avoid it and tell your doctor.
Report any unusual or severe symptoms to your doctor and follow any other advice given by him.

M.A.O.I. | Prepared by The Pharmaceutical Society and the British Medical Association on behalf of the Health Departments of the United Kingdom.

Printed in UK for HMSO D8919816 5/85 12773   33383

Figure 8 *Advice to patients prescribed a monoamine oxidase inhibitor*

Anxiety, hypochondriacal symptoms, lethargy and fatigue are prominent symptoms whereas self-blame and guilt are uncommon.

It is necessary to give these drugs in sufficient dosage for at least six weeks before clinical response can be judged. The recommended dose of phenelzine (Nardil) is 60–90 mg daily given in divided doses; of tranylcypromine (Parnate) it is 20–40 mg daily, and of isocarboxazid (Marplan) it is 30–50 mg. Tranylcypromine has a greater intrinsic stimulant action than the hydrazine MAOI phenelzine and isocarboxazid. Hydrazines are thought to be metabolised by acetylation. An individual's acetylator status is genetically determined, and there is some evidence to show that fast acetylators do less well than slow acetylators. If adequate dosage is achieved acetylator status appears to make less difference.

The observation that tyramine-containing foods such as cheese, broad beans and meat extracts can cause severe hypertensive reactions in patients taking MAOI was another factor weighing against their use. All patients prescribed these drugs must be told in detail which foods they should not eat; usually they are given a card listing them at the time the drug is dispensed (see Figure 8). Cough and cold remedies containing sympathomimetic constituents must also be avoided. Provided these simple precautions are taken there is little risk of untoward reaction.

Combining a tricyclic MARI with a MAOI does not bestow any therapeutic advantage; furthermore, it increases the occurrence of weight gain, orthostatic hypotension and impotence. Fatal reactions have rarely occurred, usually in the context of an overdose. It is generally recommended that tricyclic MARI should be withheld for at least 14 days after stopping treatment with MAOI. When given alone MAOI are prone to cause postural hypotension, sleep disturbance and weight gain. MAOI are not cardiotoxic, nor do they have any anticholinergic activity. Both the selective MAO-A inhibitor clorgyline and the MAO-B inhibitor selegiline (see page 154) are likely to cause the 'cheese reaction' at clinically effective dosage, and neither has been shown to possess any significant advantage over the standard MAOI. The deleterious effects on sleep can be minimised by appropriately adjusting the time of administration. Phenelzine has been noted to impair sexual function.

4 Other drugs

L-tryptophan (Optimax), the amino-acid precursor of 5–HT, given at a dose of 1–2 g three times daily has been shown to be more effective than placebo in the treatment of depressive syndromes in the context of both hospital and family practice. The efficacy of L-tryptophan in mild to moderate depression appears similar to that of the standard tricyclic MARI amitriptyline with a combination of the two drugs leading to greater symptomatic relief than either given alone. Side effects are few; they include gastrointestinal symptoms, drowsiness and headache.

Flupenthixol (Fluanxol), a dopamine (DA) receptor blocking drug widely used in the management of chronic schizophrenia (see chapter 6), has been shown to be equal in efficacy to standard antidepressants when given to depressed patients at a dose of 1 mg daily. In common with the other DA blockers there is a risk of extrapyramidal side effects developing. Flupenthixol is particularly useful in the management of patients who repeatedly commit suicidal acts.

Bromocriptine (Parlodel), a DA receptor agonist, has also been found equivalent to a standard antidepressant drug in the treatment of depressive illness, at a daily dose of 10–50 mg. It is necessary to increase the dose of bromocriptine gradually in order to minimise the risk of nausea and dizziness. There is preliminary evidence to suggest that bromocriptine is particularly effective in bipolar depression; if confirmed, this finding is consistent with the view that bipolar depression is neurochemically distinct from unipolar illness (see page 147).

Lithium, a drug widely used in the treatment of mania (see below), has also been shown to be effective in the treatment of depression.

Alprazolam (Xanex), a triazalobenzodiazepine derivative, when given at a dose of 1 mg three times daily was found to be significantly more effective than placebo and equivalent to standard tricyclic MARI in the treatment of depressed out-patients. This held true even for the more severely depressed patients (major depressive episode with melancholia). Alprazolam caused fewer untoward side effects than the comparison drug.

All are equally effective. Among those currently available, imipramine, amitriptyline, doxepin and dothiepin have stood the test of time, and of these dothiepin is likely to cause fewer anticholinergic side effects.

Where there is marked agitation and restlessness, a more sedative antidepressant such as amitriptyline, doxepin or mianserin given as a single dose at night is preferable, but day-time sedation may prove troublesome, particularly with mianserin. Alprazolam might prove a useful alternative, although as with any benzo-diazepine there is the potential problem of physical dependence developing (see chapter 8).

5   *ECT*   A number of double-blind clinical trials have recently been conducted in which the effects of standard ECT treatment were compared to 'placebo' ECT in which the procedure was identical apart from the passage of current through the electrodes; both groups of patients received a general anaesthetic and a muscle relaxant. The results of these studies generally support the view that ECT is an effective treatment for severe depressive illness, especially for patients suffering from delusional (psychotic) depression.

Choice of treatment

For most cases of depressive illness (major depressive episode), treatment with one of the standard tricyclic MARI antidepressants should be started as soon as the diagnosis has been established.

While there are also a variety of mixtures combining an antidepressant with an anxiolytic sedative (amitriptyline with chlordiazepoxide [Limbitrol]; amitriptyline with perphenazine [Triptafen]; nortriptyline with perphenazine [Motival]; imipramine with promazine), we would not recommend their use. If the addition of an anxiolytic sedative is thought necessary then one of the benzodiazepine group of drugs (see chapter 8) can be prescribed as required, allowing a greater flexibility of dosage. Patients who fall into the category of neurotic or atypical depression, in whom hypochrondriacal symptoms or phobic anxiety are prominent, may respond better to an MAOI such as phenelzine, although it is usual to commence with a MARI and switch over to a MAOI only if the first line of treatment proves unsuccessful.

In psychotic depression, with accompanying morbid delusions, antidepressant drugs are often ineffective. If this proves to be the case then ECT should be considered. The same applies when severe psychomotor retardation prevents adequate hydration and nutrition.

Another treatment strategy for delusional depression is the addition of an antipsychotic drug; the combination of antidepressant plus antipsychotic has been found to be superior to either type of drug given alone. Once a patient has responded satisfactorily to treatment with an antidepressant or to ECT he or she should be maintained on an antidepressant drug for some six months after recovery as stopping treatment earlier greatly increases the risk of relapse.

It is most important when stopping treatment with an antidepressant drug to do it slowly. Abrupt cessation can lead to withdrawal symptoms which include gastrointestinal symptoms, anxiety, restlessness and insomnia, and occasionally extra-pyramidal symptoms. These are thought to result from cholinergic overactivity following the removal of blockade of muscarinic receptors. Occasionally a manic syndrome may appear.

A proportion of patients with depressive illness will fail to respond to antidepressant drugs, even when given in adequate dosage, or to ECT. This situation is often referred to as 'resistant depression'. In such cases adding lithium to the pre-existing antidepressant drug may effect recovery. Other drug combinations which have been found useful in resistant depression include l-tryptophan with lithium plus clomipramine *or* phenelzine.

For the management of depression in the elderly see chapter 13.

Therapeutic drug monitoring in depression

Steady-state plasma levels of antidepressive drugs display 20–30 fold interpatient differences. This may be due not only to differences in rates of drug metabolism but also to poor patient compliance (see page 89), because studies have shown that as many as 50 per cent of patients given these drugs have stopped taking them within a few weeks of their being prescribed.

Routine measurement of plasma drug concentrations is only of value if there is a close relationship between them and therapeutic or toxicological effects. For most antidepressive drugs this has not been established. There is, however, a consensus of studies suggesting that the therapeutic effect of nortriptyline is best seen in patients with plasma levels in the range 50–150 μg/l. There is also evidence in patients treated with amitriptyline that levels of parent drug and metabolite (amitriptyline plus nortriptyline) of 100–200 μg/l are associated with a better response compared with patients outside this range.

There are a variety of analytical methods available for assaying plasma drug levels but none can yet be considered satisfactory or economical for routine use. In addition, studies have shown a great variety in performance between laboratories carrying out these assays, even when claiming to use the same techniques, and an external quality control scheme is therefore essential to ensure comparability of results between different laboratories. It is probable, however, that therapeutic drug monitoring will prove of value in improving care of patients treated with nortriptyline and amitriptyline when sensitive, reliable and cheap analytical methods are available. Indications for such monitoring include:

1 elderly patients, in whom there seems to be increased variability of plasma levels and greater vulnerability to adverse effects;
2 patients with heart disease, because of the cardiotoxic effects of monoamine-reuptake inhibiting drugs;

3 patients who fail to respond to treatment with standard doses in whom non-compliance or rapid drug clearance is suspected;

4 patients who develop adverse effects on modest drug dosage, in whom reduced clearance leading to unexpectedly high plasma levels must be distinguished from an unusual sensitivity of the patient to the drug.

Mania

1 *Antipsychotic drugs* The severely manic patient, with his non-stop activity, constant pressure of talk, bellicose self-confidence and inability to focus on any activity for more than a moment, will nearly always require urgent treatment, preferably in hospital. The neuroleptic drugs (see chapter 6), particularly the phenothiazine compound chlorpromazine (Largactil, Thorazine), the butyro-phenone, haloperidol (Serenace, Haldol) and the diphenylbutyl-piperidine compound, pimozide (Orap) have proved to be very effective in the treatment of mania.

Initially, if the patient is unwilling to take oral medication, intramuscular administration of some 250–500 mg chlorpromazine or 10–30 mg haloperidol will be required. This may need to be repeated until the patient becomes sufficiently cooperative to take the drug orally. It is usually a matter of trial and error to determine the dose which is adequate to control the symptoms without being too sedating. For chlorpromazine it is likely to lie between 75 and 200 mg three times daily, for haloperidol to be between 5 mg and 30 mg twice daily and for pimozide 10–40 mg daily. Such high doses of neuroleptics may produce marked parkinsonian effects which can be alleviated by antiparkinsonian drugs such as benzhexol (Artane) 2–4 mg three times daily, or orphenadrine (Disipal) 50–100 mg three time daily (see chapter 6).

Medication should be continued for several weeks after the patient has returned to normal, when it can be cautiously reduced. However, should any of the signs of mania reappear, treatment will then need to be maintained at a higher dose for another period of several weeks.

2 *Lithium* It would appear from well controlled trials that lithium carbonate has a definite therapeutic effect in mania, but this usually takes about a week to appear. Because of this relatively

long delay in onset of action, lithium is not particularly useful as the sole initial treatment in the more severe cases of mania which require hospital admission. Here a drug such as haloperidol with a more rapid onset of action is required. It can, however, be given once the patient has improved sufficiently on treatment with an antipsychotic, which can then be gradually tailed off as the lithium takes effect. Lithium has qualitative advantages over neuroleptics in that it produces little sedation and fewer side effects, and therefore has better patient acceptability.

Before starting treatment with lithium, thyroid function and renal function should be tested. A suitable starting dose of lithium carbonate is 800–1200 mg daily, given in divided dosage.

Plasma levels of lithium must be monitored closely at weekly intervals to begin with, with a level of between 0.8 and 1.2 mmol/L being aimed for. A level much below this is likely to be ineffective while a higher level may produce symptoms of lithium toxicity.

Early symptoms of toxicity include a fine tremor of the hands, nausea, perhaps with vomiting, and dizziness. At the first indication of toxic symptoms it is imperative to take a blood sample to determine the plasma level as soon as possible. Further treatment will depend on the level found. If it is below 1.2 mmol/L, and the patient is not vomiting, lithium can be continued cautiously, possibly at a lower dose to minimise the untoward effects. At a plasma level of greater than 1.2 mmol/L, but below 1.7 mmol/L lithium should be withheld for at least 48 hours when it may be restarted cautiously at a lower dose after determining the plasma level. Should frank vomiting or diarrhoea occur lithium must be stopped immediately and the plasma level measured as a matter of urgency. Because vomiting (and diarrhoea) is accompanied by loss of sodium, with which lithium exchanges, it greatly increases the risk of more serious toxicity occurring. This is signalled by a coarsening of the tremor, and by the onset of ataxia and dysarthria. If unchecked it can progress to drowsiness and confusion, followed by fits, coma and, eventually, death. (For the management of lithium toxicity, see chapter 15.)

3 *Anticonvulsants* The anticonvulsant drugs carbamazepine (Tegretol), sodium valproate (Epilim) and clonazepam (Rivotril) have all been shown to be effective in the treatment of mania. Of these, carbamazepine has been the most widely studied. At a dose of 800–1600 mg daily it appears equal in efficacy to both lithium

and haloperidol, and is better tolerated than the latter because of its freedom from extrapyramidal effects. However carbamazepine is not free from side effects; it can cause ataxia, gastrointestinal disturbances and drowsiness. An erythematous rash is seen in some 5 per cent of patients on the drug and drug-induced leucopenia can prove worrying.

Prophylaxis of affective disorders

Many patients who have a depressive illness or an attack of mania give a history of previous episodes of either mania or depression. These periods of illness tend to become more frequent with time, eventually occurring once or twice a year. It would obviously be of considerable benefit to such patients if these attacks of affective disorder could be prevented.

1 *Recurrent unipolar depression*

Long-term treatment with standard tricyclic MARI antidepressants amitriptyline and imipramine has been shown in two large multi-centre trials (one in the UK and one in the USA) to reduce significantly the risk of further relapse when compared to placebo. However, despite continued antidepressant treatment, approximately two thirds of patients will relapse over the following two to three years.

Long-term maintenance treatment with lithium has also been reported to be effective in reducing relapse rates; in some trials more so than the standard antidepressant compounds. In the UK multi-centre trial, lithium was found to be equal to amitriptyline. By contrast, in the US study, lithium was found to be less effective than imipramine in preventing relapse of unipolar depression. Partly on the basis of this finding, and partly because most patients will already be receiving treatment with a MARI antidepressant for their most recent depressive illness, it is recommended that where there have been two clear-cut depressive episodes in the previous five years, long-term treatment with a MARI antidepressant drug should be maintained. How long such treatment should go on for is as yet an unresolved question; probably for at least five years in the light of present knowledge. Any reduction in dose should be gradual, and reviewed at the first sign of relapse.

2   *Bipolar depression and recurrent mania*

(a)   *Lithium*   Lithium has been shown in a large number of studies to markedly reduce the risk of recurrence of manic episodes, and of depressive episodes in the context of bipolar illness.

Although lithium significantly reduces the recurrence rate of manic depressive disorders, and reduces the severity of those attacks which do occur, it is by no means always successful. In one study some 45 per cent of patients with rapidly cycling manic–depressive illness relapsed while on lithium, the majority relapsing within the first six months of treatment, in spite of adequate plasma levels. Nevertheless the success rate in preventing relapse was much greater with lithium than without. Some authorities have suggested that it is the level of lithium inside the erythrocyte, rather than the level in the plasma, which is important, and that monitoring the intra-erythrocyte lithium concentration might reduce the relapse rate still further.

The effective range of plasma levels of lithium for prophylaxis is 0.4–0.8 mmol/L. At least 12 hours should have elapsed between ingestion of the last lithium tablet taken and the blood sampling, and this should be checked with the patient on each occasion. In patients with normal renal function the biological half-life of lithium is 7–20 hours, being somewhat longer in patients with impaired renal function. During a day, therefore, lithium levels may fluctuate markedly, and it is for this reason that a fixed time must be taken for plasma level estimation.

Several preparations of lithium carbonate are available. In general there is little to choose between them; the slower release formulations such as Litarex and Liskonium do not appear to possess an advantage over the others (see page 178).

Lithium taken once daily is as effective as divided dosage, with no greater frequency of side effects, risk of toxicity or longer-term consequences.

Unwanted effects of longer-term lithium treatment include production of a reversible nephrogenic diabetes insipidus which appears to be due to inhibition of vasopressin-sensitive adenylate cyclase within the kidney with a consequent rise in serum vasopressin levels. Patients with this adverse reaction complain of thirst and polyuria which may produce disturbed sleep. Thirst also occurs without any associated polyuria, suggesting that lithium may stimulate thirst directly. Treatment consists of reduction of the dose of lithium. Permanent renal damage is unlikely to occur provided lithium toxicity is avoided.

Lithium interferes with thyroid function and can produce frank hypothyroidism with a goitre. Weight gain is seen in many patients treated with lithium but is of little significance if not associated with changes in thyroid function.

It must be remembered that symptoms of acute lithium toxicity can occur at any time during lithium prophylaxis (see page 170). Should this happen, it is imperative that lithium is discontinued immediately and the plasma level measured as a matter of urgency.

Contraindications and special precautions to lithium treatment Lithium should be administered to a patient with a history of serious renal or cardiac disease only after very careful consideration, and should only be given with great circumspection to a patient with hyperthyroidism because of its effects on thyroid function (see above). Lithium is not advised during pregnancy, particularly in the first trimester, as it has been claimed that the risk of malformation, particularly involving the cardiovascular system, is greater in children of women prescribed lithium during pregnancy than that of women not so exposed. It is probably best for a woman receiving lithium to avoid breast feeding, or to discontinue lithium if she wishes to breast feed her infant, as lithium passes into breast milk. Although old age is no contraindication to lithium treatment, progressive reduction in renal function with increasing age means that frequent monitoring of plasma level is necessary with appropriate changes in dose.

Drug interactions with lithium Sodium deficiency leads to a reduction of lithium clearance, so that a sodium-poor diet, excessive sweating and salt loss from vomiting and diarrhoea may lead to lithium intoxication. This is the basis of important interactions with diuretics which can reduce lithium clearance and lead to intoxication. Administration of thiazides may be useful for reducing the urine flow in patients with lithium-induced diabetes insipidus, but their use for this purpose must be carefully monitored in order to prevent lithium accumulation and further toxicity. Increased sodium intake, on the other hand, can lead to increased lithium excretion with a fall in plasma level.

It has been reported that lithium may potentiate muscle relaxant drugs, and anaesthetists must be aware of the patient's medication and take it into account.

(b) *Carbamazepine* Carbamazepine (Tegretol) either alone or in combination with lithium has been found to be effective in the prophylaxis of bipolar illness, especially among those who have proved to be lithium resistant. Patients described as 'rapid cyclers' have also been found to be responsive to carbamazepine. Dosage is as for mania and the side effects are the same (see page 170).

(c) *Depot antipsychotic drugs* Some patients with recurrent mania either fail to respond to, or are non-compliant with, long-term lithium or carbamazepine. Here the regular administration of a depot antipsychotic by intramuscular injection may prove effective in reducing the number of mania episodes.

Table 9 *Antidepressant drugs*

Approved name	Proprietary name	Recommended dose (daily unless stated otherwise)	Remarks
monoamine reuptake inhibiting drugs			
imipramine	Tofranil	75–200 mg	The 'standard' tricyclic compound against which others are compared. Autonomic and cardiac effects may be pronounced at higher dosage. Takes 10–14 days to act
desipramine	Pertofran Norpramine	75–200 mg	The demethylated metabolite of imipramine; no advantages over imipramine
lofepramine	Gamanil	70–140 mg	Precursor of desipramine to which it is partially metabolised. Fewer anticholinergic effects and possibly less cardiotoxic than the parent compound

Table 9   *contd.*

Approved name	Proprietary name	Recommended dose (daily unless stated otherwise)	Remarks
trimi-pramine	Surmontil	50–100 mg (as single dose before retiring)	Methylated derivative of imipramine; no obvious advantages over other tricyclics
clomi-pramine (chorimi-pramine)	Anafranil	50–150 mg (can be given as infusion)	Chloro-derivative of imipramine; no obvious advantages over imipramine. Can be given by intravenous infusion. Said to be useful in obsessional and phobic disorders
amitrip-tyline	Tryptizol Elavil	75–200 mg	Effective antidepressant with sedative properties, particularly useful in depressive illness accompanied by anxiety. Takes 10–14 days to act fully
	Lentizol	50–100 mg sustained release tablets at night	
butriptyline	Evadyne	50–150 mg	No proven advantage over amitriptyline
nor-triptyline	Aventyl	75–200 mg	Demethylated derivative of amitriptyline; no obvious advantage over amitriptyline
pro-triptyline	Concordin Triptil Vivactil	15–60 mg	Unsaturated analogue of nortriptyline; the most rapidly acting of the tricyclics. Effective within 5–10 days
doxepin	Sinequan	75–150 mg	Oxepin derivative of amitriptyline. Pronounced anxiolytic effect. Antidepressant activity equal to imipramine and amitriptyline

Table 9 *contd.*

Approved name	Proprietary name	Recommended dose (daily unless stated otherwise)	Remarks
dothiepin	Prothiaden	75–150 mg	Thiapin derivative of amitriptyline. As effective as amitriptyline with fewer autonomic side effects
iprindole	Prondol	45–90 mg	An indole central ring with imipramine side chain. As effective as imipramine and amitriptyline with fewer autonomic effects. May cause liver damage
opipramol	Insidon Ensidon	100–150 mg	Imipramine nucleus with piperazine side chain. No advantage over imipramine
dibenzepin	Noveril	240–480 mg	Structure resembles imipramine with side chain in different position. Clinically equivalent to imipramine
Newer antidepressants maprotiline	Ludiomil	50–150 mg	Rapidly acting antidepressant with relatively low incidence of anticholinergic side effects. May precipitate epileptic attack in predisposed individual
viloxazine	Vivalan	100–300 mg	Equal in efficacy to imipramine with less drowsiness and anticholinergic side effects. Prone to cause nausea
amoxapine	Demolox	120–480 mg	A tricyclic debenzoxazepine which inhibits NA reuptake and

Table 9   *contd.*

Approved name	Proprietary name	Recommended dose (daily unless stated otherwise)	Remarks
			blocks DA receptors. Can give rise to extrapyramidal symptoms and galactorrhoea. No advantage over standard antidepressants
mianserin	Bolvidon Norval	30–120 mg	Equal in efficacy to amitriptyline with virtually no anticholinergic side effects, and less danger of cardiotoxicity. Can cause drowsiness
trazodone	Molipaxin	100–300 mg	Equal in efficacy to amitriptyline with less anticholinergic and cardiotoxic properties
fluvoxamine	Faverin	100–200mg	5–HT reuptake inhibitors with no anticholinergic or cardiotoxic effects.
fluoxetine	Elatine	20mg	May cause gastrointestinal symptoms. Equal in efficacy to other antidepressants.
Monoamine oxidase inhibitors 1 *hydrazines* phenelzine iso- carboxazid iproniazid 2 *non-hydrazines*	 Nardil Marplan Marsilid	 30–60 mg 20–40 mg 50–75 mg	Little convincing evidence of efficacy in depressive illness, although certain patients respond well. All MAOI can cause severe hypertensive reaction with tyramine-containing foods (e.g. cheese), sympathomimetic amines and tricyclic antidepressants. Also potentiate action of pethidine and alcohol. May cause liver damage. Of some value in

Table 9 *contd.*

Approved name	Proprietary name	Recommended dose (daily unless stated otherwise)	Remarks
tranyl-cypromine	Parnate	20–40 mg	management of phobic disorders. Maybe genetically determined slow acetylators respond best to phenelzine due to reduced rate of metabolism of the drug
Monoamine precursors			
l-tryptophan	Optimax	1–2 g	Effective in mild to moderate depression. May enhance efficacy of MAOI. Useful in combination with MAOI or MARI in resistant depression. Taken after meals to lessen risk of gastrointestinal symptoms
Lithium preparations			
lithium carbonate	Camcolit Liskonium Priadel Phasal	Dose to be adjusted to produce blood level of 0.6 to 1.2 mmol/L	These differ in pharmacokinetic profiles. Although Camcolit and Priadel are more rapidly absorbed and eliminated than Liskonium, there is little difference clinically. All three can be given once daily. Absorption of Phasal is inconsistent
lithium citrate	Litarex	Dose to be adjusted to produce blood level of 0.6 to 1.2 mmol/L	A slow-release formulation which is similar clinically to lithium carbonate

Suggestions for further reading

Biological basis of affective disorders

CALLOWAY, S. P., DOLAN, R. J., FONAGY, O., DE SOUZA, V. F. A., and WAKELING, A., 'Endocrine changes and clinical profiles in depression', *Psychological Medicine*, vol. 14, 1984, pp. 749–66.

CHECKLEY, S. A., 'Biological markers in depression', in *Recent Advances in Clinical Psychiatry*, vol. 5, ed. K. Granville-Grossman, Churchill Livingstone, Edinburgh, 1985, pp. 201–44.

DEAKIN, J. F. W., *The Biology of Depression*, Gaskell, London, 1986.

HENINGER, G. R., CHARNEY, D. S., and STERNBERG, D. E., 'Serotonergic function in depression', *Archives of General Psychiatry*, vol. 41, 1984, pp. 398–402.

SILVERSTONE, T., and COOKSON, J., 'The biology of mania', in *Recent Advances in Clinical Psychiatry*, vol. 4, ed. K. Granville-Grossman, Churchill Livingstone, Edinburgh, 1982, pp. 201–41.

ZIS, A. P., and GOODWIN, F. K., 'The amine hypothesis', in *Handbook of Affective Disorders*, ed. E. S. Paykel, Churchill Livingstone, Edinburgh, 1982, pp. 175–90.

Pharmacology of antidepressant drugs

ALEXANDERSON, B., and SJOQVIST, F., 'Individual differences in the pharmacokinetics of non-methylated tricyclic antidepressants: role of genetic and environmental factors and clinical importance', *Annals of the New York Academy of Science*, vol. 179, 1971, pp. 1739–51.

CACCIA, S., and FONG, M. H., 'Kinetics and distribution of the β-adrenergic agonist salbutamol in rat brain', *Journal of Pharmacy and Pharmacology*, vol. 36, 1984, pp. 200–2.

GHOSE, K., COPPEN, A., and TURNER, P., 'Autonomic actions and interactions of mianserin hydrochloride and amitriptyline in patients with depressive illness', *Psychopharmacology*, vol. 49, 1976, pp. 201–4.

GHOSE, K., GIFFORD, L. A., TURNER, P., and LEIGHTON, M., 'Studies of the interaction of desmethylimipramine with tyramine in man, after a single oral dose, and its correlation with plasma concentrations', *British Journal of Clinical Pharmacology*, vol. 3, 1976, pp. 334–7.

NYBACK, H. V., WALTERS, J. R., AGHAJANIAN, G. K., and ROTH, R. H., 'Tricyclic antidepressants: effects on the firing rate of brain noradrenergic neurons', *European Journal of Pharmacology*, vol. 32, 1975, pp. 302–12.

STAHL, S. M., 'Serotonin agonists and beta-adrenergic agonists as a treatment for depressive disorder: a direct clinical application', *Psychopharmacology Bulletin*, vol. 12, 1985, pp. 43–7.

TRENCHARD, A., TURNER, P., PARE, C. M. B., and HILLS, M., 'The effects of protriptyline and clomipramine *in vitro* on the uptake of 5–hydroxy-tryptamine and dopamine in human platelet-rich plasma', *Psychopharmacologia*, vol. 43, 1975, pp. 89–93.

Antidepressants

AARONS, S. F., MANN, J. J., BROWN, R. P., YOUNG, R. G., and FRANCES, A., 'Antidepressant efficiency of L-deprenyl; clinical and biochemical correlates', in *Clinical and Pharmacological Studies in Psychiatric Disorders*, ed. G. D. Burrows, T. R. Norman and L. Dennerstein, John Libbey, London, 1985, pp. 33–6.

ASBERG, M., and SJOQVIST, F., 'Therapeutic monitoring of tricyclic antidepressants – clinical aspects', in *Therapeutic Drug Monitoring*, ed. A. Richens and V. Marks, Churchill Livingstone, Edinburgh, 1981, pp. 224–38.

BRAITHWAITE, R., 'Tricyclic antidepressants: analytical techniques', in *Therapeutic Drug Monitoring*, ed. A. Richens and V. Marks, Churchill Livingstone, Edinburgh, 1981, pp. 239–54.

JONES, S., and TURNER, P., 'An external quality control scheme for tricyclic antidepressants', *Postgraduate Medical Journal*, vol. 56 (Suppl), 1980, pp. 94–8.

NEIS, A., and ROBINSON, D. S., 'Monoamine oxidase inhibitors', in *Handbook of Affective Disorders*, ed. E. S. Paykel, Churchill Livingstone, Edinburgh, 1982, pp. 246–61.

PARE, C, M. B., 'The present status of monoamine oxidase inhibitors', *British Journal of Psychiatry*, vol. 146, 1985, pp. 576–84.

PAYKEL, E. S., 'How effective are antidepressants?' in *Psychopharmacology: Recent Advances and Future Prospects*, ed. S. D. Iversen, Oxford University Press, Oxford, 1985, pp. 3–13.

PINDER, R. M., 'α_2-adrenoceptor antagonists as antidepressants', *Drugs of the Future*, vol. 10, 1985, pp. 29–41.

POTTER, W. Z., 'Psychotherapeutic drugs and biogenic amines: current concepts and therapeutic implications', *Drugs*, vol. 28, 1984, pp. 124–43.

PRIEN, R. E. (ed.), 'Workshop report – antidepressant drug therapy: the role of the new antidepressants', *Psychopharmacology Bulletin*, vol. 20, 1984, pp. 209–302.

SCHMIDT, L. G., GROHMANN, R., MULLER-OERLINGHAUSEN, O., OCHSENFAHRT, H., and SCHONHOFER, P. S., 'Adverse drug reactions to first and second generation antidepressants', *British Journal of Psychiatry*, vol. 148, 1986, pp. 38–43.

ECT

JOHNSTONE, E. C., 'The Northwick Park ECT Trial', *Lancet*, vol. 11, 1980, pp. 1317–20.

PALMER, R. L., *Electroconvulsive Therapy*, Oxford University Press, 1981.

SLADE, A. P., and CHECKLEY, S. A., 'A neuroendocrine study of the mechanism of action of ECT', *British Journal of Psychiatry*, vol. 137, 1980, pp. 217–21.

WEST, E. D., 'ECT in depression: a double-blind controlled trial', *British Medical Journal*, vol. 282, 1981, pp. 355–7.

Treatment of mania

BROWN, D., SILVERSTONE, T., and COOKSON, J., 'Carbamazepine compared to haloperidol in acute mania' (in preparation).

DOSE, M., EMRICH, H. M., CORDING-TOMMEL, C., and VON ZERSSEN, D., 'Antimanic properties of the calcium antagonist verapamil', in *Clinical and Pharmacological Studies in Psychiatric Disorders*, ed. G. D. Burrows, T. R. Norman and L. Dennerstein, John Libbey, London, 1985, pp. 96–100.

SILVERSTONE, T., 'Dopamine in manic depressive illness', *Journal of Affective Disorders*, vol. 8, 1985, pp. 225–31.

TYRER, S. P., 'Lithium in the treatment of mania', *Journal of Affective Disorders*, vol. 8, 1985, pp. 251–7.

Prophylaxis of affective disorder

GLEN, A. I. M., JOHNSON, A. L., and SHEPHERD, M., 'Continuation therapy with lithium and amitriptyline in unipolar depressive illness', *Psychological Medicine*, vol. 14, 1984, pp. 37–50.

POST, R. M., UHDE, T. W., BALLENGER, J. C., and SQUILLACE, K. M., 'Prophylactic efficacy of carbamazepine in manic–depressive illness', *American Journal of Psychiatry*, vol. 140, 1983, pp. 1602–4.

PRIEN, R. F., KUPFER, D. J., MANSKY, P. A., SMALL, J. G., TUASON, V. B., VOSS, C. B., and JOHNSON, W. E., 'Drug therapy in the prevention of recurrences in unipolar and bipolar affective disorders', *Archives of General Psychiatry*, vol. 41, 1984, pp. 1096–104.

SHUKLA, S., COOKE, B. L., and MILLER, M. G., 'Lithium-carbamazepine versus lithium-neuroleptic prophylaxis in bipolar illness', *Journal of Affective Disorders*, vol. 9, 1985, pp. 219–22.

Anxiety

8

Anxiety is an inevitable by-product of the process by which a person learns to become a member of society. . . . The fact that the human being can experience fear permits this learning to take place. In the process anxiety arises.

Levitt

Introduction

Anxiety and fear play a vital role in all human societies. To feel anxious in the face of a threatening stimulus is both normal and appropriate; it is only when the anxiety becomes so severe as to be incapacitating, or arises without reasonable cause, that clinical intervention is indicated. Unfortunately this occurs all too frequently. In a large epidemiological survey in the London area it was found that 14 per cent of the population at risk consulted the doctor at least once during the course of a year for symptoms which were a reflection of underlying anxiety. A Scandinavian study revealed that one third of the adult population had overt symptoms of anxiety, nervousness or tension; 5 per cent had symptoms severe enough to warrant the diagnosis of an anxiety state.

Reflecting this widespread prevalence of anxiety is the large number of prescriptions issued for anxiolytic/sedative drugs throughout the developed world. In the UK a recent survey revealed that 3 per cent of adults (representing 1.25 million people) had taken a benzodiazepine regularly for at least one year (see chapter 5).

Psychopathology

Within the overall spectrum of anxiety disorders a number of clinical subcategories have been delineated and defined. These include anxiety states, panic attacks, phobias and obsessive compulsive disorder.

1 *Anxiety states (*DSM III *– generalised anxiety disorder)*

This is characterised by generalised and persistant feelings of anxiety and foreboding, increased distractability and irritability, and frequently present are an impairment of concentration and a sleep disturbance. Common autonomic accompaniments (see below) are palmar sweating, palpitations, tremulousness, dry mouth and flushing. Patients may also experience a wide variety of other somatic symptoms, the physiological basis of which is obscure. These can include light-headedness, paraesthesiae, hot or cold spells, 'butterfly stomach', frequency of micturition and/or defaecation, and a lump in the throat.

2 *Panic attacks (*DSM III *– panic disorder)*

This condition is characterised by recurrent attacks of panic, amounting at times to frank terror, often accompanied by an inexplicable but overwhelming sensation of imminent death. These attacks typically arise without warning and with no obvious precipitant. Further convincing the patient that the worst is about to happen are the frequent sensations of choking and smothering together with a rapid tachycardia and profuse sweating. There is a pronounced tendency to overbreathe which in turn brings on paraesthesiae, and dizziness.

3 *Phobias and situational anxiety (*DSM III *– phobic disorders)*

Phobias can be regarded as the irrational avoidance of a particular set of situations or objects due to an exaggerated fear of them. The fear often arises out of a learned experience. The phobic disorders are usually classified as falling into one of three categories, simple phobias, social phobias and agoraphobia.

(a) *Simple phobias* Avoidance of particular objects (frequently a particular type of animal, e.g. spiders, snakes) or situations (e.g. heights).

(b) *Social phobias* Avoidance of social situations in which the individual is exposed to the scrutiny of others (e.g. eating in public).

(c) *Agoraphobia* This is the most pervasive and restricting form of phobic disorder in which the sufferer finds great difficulty in leaving the security of his or her own home. Crowded shopping areas and bustling streets are particularly avoided. A companion may be required for even the shortest forays into the world outside; with some patients becoming completely housebound. There is usually a history of a life-long tendency to experience heightened anxiety.

4   *Obsessive–compulsive disorder*

In this condition patients are plagued by recurrent thoughts and preoccupied by the need to perform recurrent acts which they recognise as unnecessary, but which they are powerless to resist because of the resultant fear that some disaster will occur should they desist.

Psychophysiology

The subjective awareness of anxiety and fear is associated with general 'arousal' of the central nervous system plus peripheral autonomic discharge. Stimuli which are seen as threatening produce activation of the reticular activating system (RAS) in the brain stem, probably via corticofugal pathways passing down from the cerebral cortex to the reticular formation, the cortex classifying the particular stimuli as being threatening or not. It is likely that the cerebral cortex and the RAS together constitute a feedback-control system maintaining an optimal arousal level. Through this system when cortical activity is great the RAS activity is inhibited, thereby preventing too great an arousal level. Should this inhibition of the RAS break down then the cortical activity may continue unchecked, leading to a state of incapacitating anxiety.

In addition other areas of the brain are clearly involved in the pathogenesis of anxiety, particularly the structures grouped in the limbic system, including the amygdala and the hippocampus, together with areas in the hypothalamus. Stimulation of the posterior hypothalamus in laboratory animals leads to behaviour suggestive of a panic reaction; stimulation of the same area in humans is reported as being most unpleasant. It is believed that the hypothalamic centres, which probably regulate the autonomic discharge seen in anxiety, are themselves under the control of the hippocampus and amygdala; on the one hand the amygdala increases, and on the other the hippocampus and septal region inhibits the hypothalamic response to threatening stimuli.

It has been found that stimulation of the centro-medial hypothalamus in a normally placid cat will generate aggressive behaviour which can be considerably modified by simultaneous stimulation of the amygdala. Furthermore, such electrical stimulation of the amygdala produces a rapid rise in 17-hydroxycorticosteroids presumably by increasing ACTH production via the hypothalamic pituitary axis.

Additional experimental evidence for the view that these regions of the brain are important in the production of anxiety comes from studies using implanted electrodes. When electrodes are placed in certain areas of the brain of a rat (e.g. the septal region and the lateral hypothalamus), and the animal can turn on the current by pressing a lever with its foot (self-stimulation), it is repeatedly found that the rat will continuously stimulate itself in this way for hours at a time, ignoring food and water. If an animal has been trained to expect a shock on hearing a click it will normally cower in a corner of its cage when the click sounds. If however it is able to self-stimulate its septal area it will ignore the sound of the click and even when the electric shock is applied to its feet it will not show any sign of a fear reaction; it just keeps on self-stimulating.

The hippocampal–amygdala system is in turn regulated by the cerebral cortex which, as we have seen, is modulated by the RAS through a feedback loop.

Histochemical studies have shown that the neurones of the lower brain stem, where the RAS is situated, contain noradrenaline (NA) and dopamine (DA). These particular neurones have widespread synaptic connections with the limbic system and it has been postulated that NA may act as the transmitter in the system underlying anxiety responses, particularly as the NA levels in NA cells rise during the performance of a conditioned avoidance response. In addition to the NA cells in the lower brain stem there are others projecting to the lateral hypothalamus and the hippocampus which synthesise 5-hydroxytryptamine (5–HT). It could be that these two cell types themselves act reciprocally, the

NA cell system increasing the anxiety response and the 5–HT cell system reducing it. In keeping with this hypothesis is the finding that members of the benzodiazepine group of drugs (see below) which are effective in the treatment of anxiety, can increase brain 5–HT levels, possibly by promoting the release of gamma-aminobutyric acid (GABA), a neurotransmitter which probably inhibits noradrenergic activity.

Whatever the central mechanism involved, the subjective experience of anxiety is usually accompanied by widespread sympathetic discharge together with a steep rise in circulating catecholamines. The particular autonomic changes which have been most studied are those occurring in the cardiovascular system and those in the palmar sweat glands.

Increased anxiety has long been known to be associated with a quickening of the heart. Measurements of peripheral blood flow, using venous occlusion plethysmography, have demonstrated that when an individual is anxious his forearm blood flow also increases. These autonomic responses can reinforce the central awareness of anxiety and thus compound the symptoms' severity; such cardiovascular concomitants often make the patient seek medical advice.

The palmar sweat glands, which have little thermoregulatory function, are innervated by the sympathetic nervous system but, unlike the rest of this system, are cholinergic rather than adrenergic. Thus drugs blocking adrenergic responses (i.e. the beta-adrenergic blockers – see below) do not affect increased palmar sweating although they can effectively reduce psychogenic tachycardia. The level of palmar sweating determines the electrical resistance of the palmar skin. When sweating is marked, resistance is low, and vice versa. This phenomenon is the basis of the so-called psychogalvanic response (see chapter 4) which has proved to be a most useful physiological variable with which to compare states of psychological arousal.

The autonomic accompaniments of anxiety are so pervasive that at one time it was thought that they, rather than any central phenomena, actually caused the anxiety. This view was shown to be erroneous by Cannon and it came to be accepted that the experience of anxiety was entirely dependent on the central state, with little reference to what was occurring peripherally.

This was perhaps too great a swing of the pendulum. Some patients certainly find that the degree of anxiety which they experience is modulated by their awareness of autonomic symptoms, particularly tachycardia. For them simple reduction of this tachycardia by peripheral beta-adrenergic receptor blockade with a drug such as propranolol affords significant symptomatic relief. However, this applies to only a minority of anxious patients; most require lowering of their state of heightened arousal by a centrally acting compound.

Pharmacology of antianxiety drugs

Drugs used in the treatment of anxiety states may be divided broadly into two groups, namely those which act primarily on the central nervous system and those which block peripheral autonomic receptors.

Centrally acting drugs

1   *Benzodiazepine drugs*   These have established themselves as the most widely used antianxiety drugs. Chlordiazepoxide was first marketed in the mid-1960s and rapidly became popular despite its relatively mild antianxiety activity. It was followed by diazepam, nitrazepam, medazepam, oxazepam, lorazepam, temazepam, ketazolam and potassium clorazepate. These compounds are 1:4 benzodiazepines and are closely related metabolically. Figure 9 shows that the major metabolite of diazepam is N-desmethyldiazepam (nordiazepam) which is pharmacologically active. Metabolites of diazepam and nordiazepam are temazepam and oxazepam respectively, which themselves are marketed compounds and lack active metabolites. Another marketed compound, potassium clorazepate, is a pro-drug metabolised to nordiazepam, and marketed medazepam is converted to diazepam. Some investigators have questioned whether these various marketed drugs differ significantly from one another in view of their close metabolic interrelationships.

Mechanism of action   Benzodiazepines appear to bind to specific receptors on neuronal cell membranes, resulting in a facilitation of the effects of the inhibitory transmitter GABA. These receptors are found in high concentration in the cerebral cortex, midbrain and limbic structures. An endogenous ligand has been sought for

187

CLINICAL APPLICATIONS

benzodiazepine receptors analogous to β-endorphin for opiate receptors (page 17).

It looks as if benzodiazepine-GABA receptor complexes at various different brain sites mediate the antianxiety, anticonvulsant, muscle relaxant and hypnotic effects of this group of drugs. These complexes are in turn influenced by 5–HT pathways coming from the raphé nuclei and by noradrenergic pathways from the locus coeruleus. Benzodiazepine receptor antagonists have been developed which inhibit or reverse the action of benzodiazepines in the CNS. These have a potential application in anaesthetic practice and in the management of overdose (see chapter 15). Other drugs acting on these receptors, in a manner different from the benzodiazepines, are called 'inverse agonists'; in contrast to the benzodiazepines they promote anxiety rather than alleviate it. One such group of drugs are the beta-carbolines (see below).

Pharmacokinetics   As might be expected, those 1:4-benzodiazepines that have the common major metabolite nordiazepam, namely diazepam, medazepam, ketazolam and clorazepate, are indistinguishable because the metabolite is active pharmacologically and has a longer half-life than those of the parent compounds (Table 10). This complicates their pharmacokinetic profiles, because it means that steady-state levels of the parent drugs will be reached before that of nordiazepam, which will continue to accumulate in the plasma and tissues while the drug continues to be administered. These four compounds, therefore, are long-acting and more suitable as antianxiety rather than hypnotic agents.

Table 10 *Elimination half-lives of some benzodiazepine drugs and their important metabolites in man*

Parent drug	Half-life (hours)	Important metabolite	Half-life (hours)
Alprazolam	10–20	None	
Bromazepam	10–29		
Chlordiazepoxide	10–20	N-desmethyl chlordiazepoxide	10–30
Clobazam	10–30	N-desmethyl clobazam	30–50

188

Table 10   *cont.*

Parent drug	Half-life (hours)	Important metabolite	Half-life (hours)
Clorazepate	Mainly hydrolysed before absorption	N-desmethyl-diazepam	50–100
Diazepam	20–45	N-desmethyl-diazepam	50–100
Flunitrazepam	9–31		
Flurazepam	Very short	N-desmethyl flurazepam	50–100
Ketazolam	Very short	N-desmethyl diazepam	50–100
Loprazolam	7–8	None	
Lorazepam	10–20	None	
Lormetazepam	9–15	None	
Medazepam	short	Diazepam N-desmethyl-diazepam	20–45 50–100
Midazolam	1.3–3	None	
Nitrazepam	20–40	None	
Oxazepam	10–20	None	
Prazepam	Rapidly transformed	N-desmethyl-diazepam	50–100
Temazepam	5–9	None	
Triazolam	2–4	7-α-hydroxy-derivative	3–6

CLINICAL APPLICATIONS

Oxazepam, temazepam and lorazepam do not have important active metabolites, and their half-lives are shorter. Temazepam is marketed as a short-acting hypnotic; oxazepam penetrates the blood–brain barrier more slowly and is less suitable for this purpose.

Triazolam is a benzodiazepine derivative with a triazole structure, and a half-life of only 2–4 hours. Its active metabolite also has a short half-life and triazolam is being assessed as a short-acting hypnotic drug.

Clobazam is 1:5 benzodiazepine which shows less impairment of psychomotor function for a given antianxiety effect than 1:4 benzodiazepines.

Adverse effects Overdosage with benzodiazepines, accidentally or for suicidal purposes, produces drowsiness, sleep, confusion, incoordination, muscle weakness, ataxia, diplopia and dysarthria. Serious respiratory depression seldom occurs unless there is pre-existing respiratory disease, or unless another central depressant is taken at the same time. Although relatively safe when taken alone, benzodiazepines may potentiate the central depressant effects of alcohol and barbiturate drugs and such combinations can be dangerous.

Some degree of psychomotor impairment often follows administration of therapeutic doses of benzodiazepines, and this has obvious implications for car driving or handling complex machinery (see chapter 5). Memory can also be impaired, particularly by lorazepam.

Dependence Physical dependence on benzodiazepine has been recognised as occurring much more frequently than was originally supposed with up to one third of long-term users being affected. It is characterised by a distinctive withdrawal syndrome on stopping the drug which has some of the features of a recrudescence of anxiety; thus when it occurs it frequently leads to the patient reverting to taking benzodiazepines in the mistaken belief that his or her anxiety is returning in full force. However, in contrast to what usually happens in severe generalised anxiety, the withdrawal symptoms gradually abate over the course of the next two to four weeks without further medication being required; it may take much longer in some patients for complete disappearance of withdrawal symptoms to occur. This dependence is presumably due to a gradual change in the sensitivity of the benzodiazepine sites,

190

leading to tolerance to the pharmacological effects of these drugs. It has been clearly shown that their chronic use is associated with a gradual diminution in their hypnotic and anticonvulsant effects, and this may also be true of their antianxiety activities. The withdrawal syndrome includes insomnia, anxiety, tremulousness, muscle tension, twitchings and distorted perception (such as hypersensitivity to auditory stimuli and abnormal bodily sensations); gastrointestinal symptoms are common as is depersonalisation; on occasion frank convulsions can occur. While physical dependence is most usually seen in patients who have been taking benzodiazepines for three to six months, it has been reported after as short a treatment period as one month. The dosage required is also variable, ranging upwards from 4 mg diazepam daily. Withdrawal symptoms have been observed following treatment with virtually all benzodiazepine compounds; even triazolam, with its ultra-short duration of action, may cause rebound anxiety within 24 hours. The syndrome is particularly severe when high doses have been given, for example 30 mg or more of diazepam daily. Its appearance on stopping or reducing long-term therapy has led many patients to continue unnecessary treatment. Similarly, the tolerance that may occur with repeated administration can lead to escalation of dosage above that recommended. If a benzo- diazepine drug is prescribed for anxiety, therefore, it should be given in as low a dosage and for as short a time as possible. The patient should be warned against increasing the dose without medical instruction, or abruptly discontinuing it.

The essential principle in the management of withdrawal from benzodiazepines is gradual reduction of plasma drug concentration. It is therefore advantageous to switch to a longer-acting one such as diazepam and then slowly tail off the dose over a period of weeks, titrating the rate of reduction against the patient's symptoms. Direct withdrawal from lorazepam is said to be particularly troublesome. Psychological support in the form of self- help groups may be of assistance to patients trying to wean themselves off benzodiazepines; other anxiety management tech- niques may also be beneficial. Propranolol reduces some of the somatic symptoms but is of only modest benefit overall; clonidine likewise has only a limited effect.

2 *Buspirone (Buspar)* Buspirone is a recently introduced non- benzodiazepine antianxiety drug. In contrast to the benzo-

diazepines it is non-sedative and lacks anticonvulsant and muscle-relaxant properties. Its mode of action remains obscure, although an interaction with central 5–HT systems is a possibility.

Buspirone has been shown to be useful in the treatment of anxiety when given at a daily dose of 15–30 mg, but it may take up to two weeks to become fully effective. It does not impair psychomotor function, nor does it appear to promote physical dependence; but longer-term use in a large number of patients is necessary before such a lack of dependence potential can be confidently established.

3 *Barbiturate drugs* In recent years the use of these drugs as antianxiety and hypnotic agents has reduced considerably, primarily because the ratio between the doses necessary to relieve symptoms and signs of anxiety or to induce sleep, and those which produce other evidence of central nervous depression, particularly of the respiratory centre, is small.

Apart from the dangers of overdosage, there are two other important disadvantages which barbiturates possess:

(i) a tendency to produce drug dependence
(ii) induction of liver microsomal enzymes

Therapeutic doses of barbiturate drugs are sufficient to stimulate the activity of liver microsomal enzyme systems concerned with

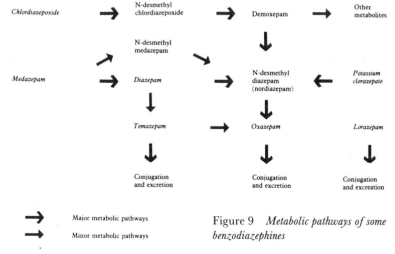

Figure 9 *Metabolic pathways of some benzodiazephines*

their own metabolism and with that of other drugs. This stimulating effect, or induction, is associated with increased liver weight, increased production of microsomal protein, and changes in the smooth membrane of the endoplasmic reticulum. Among the drugs whose half-lives are known to be reduced by treatment with barbiturate drugs are: (i) coumarin anticoagulants, leading to a reduction in their hypoprothrombinaemic effects, (ii) phenytoin, reducing its anticonvulsant effect, (iii) griseofulvin, the antifungal agent, (iv) corticosteroids and (v) oral contraceptives.

The most important of these interactions is with the coumarin drugs. It was not uncommon for a patient admitted to hospital following a myocardial infarction to be treated with a coumarin anticoagulant drug and also with a barbiturate such as pheno-barbitone to relieve anxiety and mental distress. The latter drug, by liver enzyme induction, increased the rate of hydroxylation of the coumarin drug so reducing its anticoagulant effect, which led in turn to an increase in the dose required to obtain the desired prolongation of prothrombin time. When the barbiturate drug was withdrawn, often when the patient left hospital, the microsomal enzyme activity returned to normal over a period of two or three weeks. Unless the dose of the anticoagulant drug was reduced during this period, a dangerous increase in prothrombin time might occur as its rate of metabolism returned to normal, producing a potentially dangerous haemorrhagic tendency. Benzo-diazepines do not induce liver enzymes significantly at therapeutic doses and therefore do not produce these drug interactions.

Mechanism of action The mechanism of the central nervous action of barbiturates is not fully understood. They appear to interfere with synaptic transmission at lower doses than are required to block conduction of nerve impulses along an axon. Several ways in which they influence synaptic transmission have been suggested, including decreasing release of excitatory trans-mitters, increasing release of inhibitory transmitters, decreasing sensitivity of post-synaptic receptors to excitatory transmitters, and increasing the sensitivity of post-synaptic receptors to inhibitory transmitters. At low doses the main action of barbiturates appears to be enhancement of the inhibitory synaptic mechanisms mediated by GABA. This action is quite different from that of benzo-diazepines, however, since barbiturates do not compete with diazepam for binding at specific benzodiazepine receptor sites.

4 *Propanediols* Meprobamate (Equanil), like mephenesin from which it is derived, is a skeletal muscle-relaxing compound in experimental animals, but in addition has tranquillising properties in man. It used to be a popular antianxiety drug, but since the introduction of the benzodiazepines its use has declined. Drowsiness, tolerance, dependence and hypersensitivity reactions occur frequently.

A wide variety of other centrally acting drugs have at one time or another been tried in the treatment of anxiety symptoms. While many have been shown under double-blind conditions to be more effective than placebo, few, if any, are clearly better than the benzodiazepines (see Table 11).

The sedative action of alcohol should not be forgotten in transient or mild anxiety states, particularly in elderly patients. Insomnia, restlessness and nervousness may often be allayed by the judicious use of an alcoholic beverage.

Peripherally acting drugs

Many of the manifestations of anxiety already described are probably due to an increased release of adrenaline and noradrenaline from the adrenal medulla and sympathetic nerves, and changes in urinary excretion of these amines and their metabolites have been demonstrated in patients suffering from anxiety. For this reason adrenergic blockade with drugs, such as propranolol, is effective in reducing or abolishing anxiety symptoms, particularly those which are predominantly autonomic in nature like palpitations and tremor. Relatively small doses of propranolol such as 20 to 40 mg six- or eight-hourly may be used together with small doses of a benzodiazepine drug. It must be remembered that, in some patients, bronchial asthma is a manifestation of anxiety; when this happens propranolol and other beta blockers are contraindicated.

Anxiety-inducing drugs

1 Beta-carbolines

As already stated, the beta-carbolines which act on benzodiazepine receptors as inverse agonists (i.e. in a manner opposite to that of benzodiazepines) can produce marked anxiety symptoms when given to normal subjects. This effect is attenuated by benzodiazepine receptor antagonist compounds.

2 *Alpha-2 receptor blockers*

Drugs which act by blocking alpha-2 adrenergic autoreceptors can give rise to marked anxiety in normal subjects. Included in this category are yohimbine and piperoxane. Yohimbine-induced anxiety can be countered by the alpha-2 autoreceptor agonist clonidine; the site of action of both these drugs is presumed to be the locus coeruleus, a point of origin of much of the noradrenergic innervation of many brain centres (see above). Such observations support the view that central adrenergic pathways play an important role in the pathogenesis of anxiety.

3 *Caffeine*

Caffeine, which is thought to act mainly by blocking adenosine receptors, can precipitate severe anxiety in otherwise normal subjects when taken at doses of 500 mg or more (equivalent to five cups of strong coffee). Anxiety-prone subjects are more susceptible and may experience anxiety-related symptoms at a lower dose. Thus it is important to inquire about caffeine consumption in all patients presenting with anxiety as simple reduction of caffeine intake may be sufficient to lead to significant improvement.

4 *Sodium lactate*

Infusion of sodium lactate has long been known to induce panic attacks in some normal subjects as well as in individuals prone to such attacks (see above). The site and mechanism of action of this lactate effect is unknown.

Drug treatment of anxiety

Generalised anxiety disorder

When a patient presents with either the psychological symptoms of anxiety (excessive worrying, inability to concentrate, difficulty in getting off to sleep) or its somatic accompaniments (palpitations, tension headaches, sweaty palms), the first step is to establish whether or not there is a reasonable cause for these symptoms to arise at that particular time. If so, it may be possible for the situation to be adjusted in such a way that the anxiety-provoking circumstances no longer apply.

Recognition of the underlying cause may, therefore, be itself of considerable therapeutic benefit. If, however, as is so often the case, the causative factors cannot be defined or modified, or there are no adequate grounds for the patient's symptoms, symptomatic relief is the next step. Attempts should first be made to effect this by using psychological techniques, including explanation and reassurance, supplemented when necessary with self-help literature and training in relaxation techniques. However, the symptoms may be so obtrusive as to make such an approach inappropriate as the initial treatment. In such cases it will be necessary to reduce the level of anxiety directly using drugs.

Before starting drug treatment it should be determined whether or not the patient's symptoms are but an acute episode in a normally non-anxious individual, or whether they reflect a long-standing predisposition to the development of frequent, perhaps even continuous, anxiety. In the former situation it is likely that remission will occur without any definitive therapeutic intervention. 40–50 per cent of such cases have been shown to remit spontaneously. Thus definitive treatment may not prove necessary. If drug treatment is required a benzodiazepine given for a short period (not exceeding a few weeks so as to avoid the risk of dependence) may well reduce anxiety symptoms sufficiently for the patient to cope more effectively with any associated or causal life problems, and also allow him or her to learn other strategies for dealing with stress over the longer term.

Whenever a benzodiazepine is prescribed the patient must be warned of the potential sedative effects and be cautioned against driving a motor vehicle or operating complex machinery should such effects be experienced. It is therefore wise to advise patients not to drive for a day or two after starting on a benzodiazepine so that the degree of day-time sedation can be gauged and dosage adjusted accordingly.

Whether one member of this group of drugs possesses any distinct advantages over the others is open to question. When comparisons have been made between them it has usually been on the basis of fixed dosages, so that the finding that diazepam 5 mg three times daily is more effective than chlordiazepoxide 10 mg three times daily does not necessarily imply that an increased dose of chlordiazepoxide would not be better still. The most widely prescribed benzodiazepine for the relief of anxiety is undoubtedly diazepam, and when used with due circumspection diazepam (5–20 mg daily) is a most effective antianxiety drug for the majority of patients. Overwhelming anxiety often requires larger doses, at least initially. In view of its long half-life it needs, after the first few days only, be administered on a daily basis. However, some patients prefer the flexibility which multiple dosage gives them; this may reflect the fact that the peak plasma level occurs within an hour or so after oral administration and is followed by a rapid redistribution phase in which plasma levels fall. Lorazepam, 1–2.5 mg given twice daily, in view of its shorter half-life has been found to be equally effective, but it carries a greater risk of causing dependency. Fine adjustment of dosage can often be left to the individual patient who is usually in the best position to judge the optimum dose for his symptoms. It is illogical and unnecessary to prescribe more than one benzodiazepine compound at a time. For instance, there is no justification for prescribing a short-acting benzodiazepine to relieve insomnia if the patient is already taking a longer-acting drug. The administration and dosage of the longer-acting drug should be appropriately adjusted instead. Where it is important to avoid any sedation or psychomotor impairment clobazam may have some advantage over diazepam. Buspirone, if it fulfils its early promise, should prove a valuable alternative to the benzodiazepines, particularly when rapid relief of symptoms is not an urgent clinical problem.

When there is a pronounced cardiovascular element in the symptomatology, with one of the patient's main complaints being tachycardia, it may be helpful to prescribe a beta-adrenergic blocking compound in addition to the anxiolytic sedative. Propranolol 20 to 40 mg three or four times a day has been shown to be effective; other compounds in this group like oxprenolol and sotalol may also prove of value.

Panic disorder

Imipramine, a standard tricyclic monoamine reuptake inhibitor (MARI) antidepressant drug (see chapter 7), when given at a dose of 150–300 mg daily, has been found in a number of studies to reduce significantly the frequency and severity of recurrent panic attacks, and is probably the current treatment of choice. Other MARI antidepressants appear to exert a similar therapeutic effect.

Monoamine oxidase inhibitors (MAOI) such as phenelzine (see chapter 7) have also been recommended for the management of panic attacks especially when occurring in association with phobic symptoms (see below).

Alprazolam, a triazolobenzodiazepine with antidepressant activity (see chapter 7), has also been found to be effective; but longer-term use raises the problem of physical dependence with subsequent withdrawal symptoms.

Phobic disorders

In recent years it has come to be accepted that the most effective therapeutic approach to such conditions is behaviour therapy. This 'specific desensitisation' may take the form of gradually reintroducing the patient, at first in imagination, later, in reality, to his feared situation. Another technique, 'implosion' or 'flooding', is to plunge the patient in at the deep end, as it were, by repeatedly confronting him with his most feared object or getting him to imagine himself in his most feared situation.

While there is some uncertainty whether the addition of psychotropic drugs to the behavioural approach assists in the resolution of phobic symptoms, it does appear, on balance, that the antidepressant MARI imipramine and the MAOI phenelzine, if given in sufficient dosage for a sufficiently long period of time (up to 26 weeks), can be useful adjuncts to behaviour therapy.

Obsessive–compulsive disorder

Here, too, behaviour therapy is the sheet-anchor of management. The antidepressant drug clomipramine at a dose of up to 300 mg daily has been found to be of benefit when prescribed as an adjunct to behaviour therapy, particularly when there are superimposed depressive symptoms. Such treatment is not without its problems, however. In addition to the well-recognised anticholinergic side effects associated with this type of antidepressant (see chapter 7) clomipramine is particularly prone to cause sexual difficulties leading to ejaculatory failure in men and anorgasmia in men and women.

Table 11 *Anxiolytic drugs*

Approved name	Proprietary name	Recommended dose (daily unless stated otherwise)	Remarks
benzodiazepines			
alprazolam	Xanax	1–3 mg	Triazolobenzodiazepine with antidepressant as well as anxiolytic activity
bromazepam	Lexotan	9–36 mg	Intermediate half-life with no active metabolites
chlor-diazepoxide	Librium	10–100 mg	1:4 benzodiazepines metabolised to N-desmethyldiazepam (nordiazepam). All equally effective and all have long half-lives. Can produce dependence and withdrawal symptoms
clorazepate	Tranxene	15–30 mg	
diazepam	Valium	4–60 mg	
ketazolam	Anxon	15–30 mg	
medazepam	Nobrium	10–50 mg	
lorazepam	Ativan	2–10 mg	Efficacy equal to other benzodiazepines, particularly prone to cause withdrawal symptoms on stopping
oxazepam	Serenid-D	20–90 mg	
clobazam	Frisium	20–60 mg	Structurally a 1:5 benzodiazepine. Possibly less psychomotor impairment
Other antianxiety drugs			
buspirone	Buspar	15–30 mg	Little if any sedative action or psychomotor impairment. Can take up to 2 weeks for full effect
meprobamate	Miltown Equanil	400–2400 mg	Rather weak anxiolytics. Developed from muscle-relaxants

Suggestions for further reading

General

DOROW, R., 'Anxiety and its generation by pharmacological means', in *Psychopharmacology: Recent Advances and Future Prospects*, ed. S. D. Iversen, Oxford University Press, Oxford, 1985.

GRAY, J. A., 'The neuropsychology of anxiety', *Behaviour and Brain Science*, vol. 5, 1982, pp. 469–534.

Benzodiazepines

CATALAN, J., and GATH, D. H., 'Benzodiazepines in general practice: time for a decision', *British Medical Journal*, vol. 290, 1985, pp. 1374–6.

HALLSTROM, C., 'Benzodiazepines: clinical practice and central mechanisms', in *Recent Advances in Clinical Psychiatry*, vol. 5, ed. K. Granville-Grossman, Churchill Livingstone, Edinburgh, 1985, pp. 143–60.

HIGGETT, A. C., LADER, M. H., and FONAGY, P., 'Clinical management of benzodiazepine dependence', *British Medical Journal*, vol. 291, 1985, pp. 688–90.

IVERSEN, S. D., 'Where in the central nervous system do benzodiazepines act?' in *Psychopharmacology: Recent Advances and Future Prospects*, ed. S. D. Iversen, Oxford University Press, Oxford, 1985, pp. 75–88.

RICHENS, A., and GRIFFITHS, A. M., 'Pharmacokinetic and pharmacodynamic relationships with benzodiazepines', in *Psychopharmacology: Recent Advances and Future Prospects*, ed. S. D. Iversen, Oxford University Press, Oxford, 1985, pp. 89–99.

Other drug treatments

GOA, K. L., and WARD, A., 'Buspirone', *Drugs*, vol. 32, 1986, pp. 114–29.

JUDD, F. K., NORMAN, T. R., and BURROWS, G. D., 'Pharmacological treatment of panic disorders', *International Clinical Psychopharmacology*, vol. 1, 1986, pp. 3–16.

LELLIOTT, P. T., and MONTEIRO, W. D., 'Drug treatment of obsessive–compulsive disorder', *Drugs*, vol. 31, 1986, pp. 75–80.

MATUZAR, W., and GLASS, R. M., 'Treatment of agoraphobia and panic attacks', *Archives of General Psychiatry*, vol. 40, 1983, pp. 220–2.

PEET, M., and ALI, S., 'Propranolol and atenolol in the treatment of anxiety', *International Clinical Psychopharmacology*, vol. 1, 1986, pp. 314–19.

Organic psychiatric syndromes

9

The term 'organic psychiatric syndromes' refers to those conditions in which there is a disturbance of psychological function due to a definite physical cause. That is not to say that other psychiatric conditions, such as schizophrenia or mania, are not primarily due to physical causes; they may well be. It is just that we have not yet determined with any confidence what they are (see chapters 6 and 7). In the case of the organic psychiatric syndromes, the disruption of cerebral function leading to the psychological disturbance may either be temporary (acute) or permanent (chronic).

Such phenomena as metabolic upsets, anoxia, hypoglycaemia, high fever and acute poisons frequently produce an impairment of cerebral function with an accompanying disturbance of consciousness. This gives rise to the clinical condition known as an 'acute confusional state'. Usually improvement of the underlying cause is followed promptly by amelioration of the mental state. In contrast, where the psychological impairment is due to permanent damage of the brain, as in *dementia* and the *dysmnesic syndrome* (see below), no significant spontaneous improvement can be expected.

Acute confusional state (delirium)

Whenever the level of consciousness is impaired, however slightly, there is an associated reduction in attention, with an increase in distractability. The more profound the reduction in consciousness the greater the psychological disturbance. This lessening of attention leads to a failure in grasping instructions and in registering new information. The patient thus becomes seemingly uncooperative, even truculent. In addition there may be delusions of persecution, and these, together with the restlessness and irritability which commonly occur, can make nursing difficult. Inability to register new information leads to disorientation in time and space. Such disorientation together with clouding of consciousness are cardinal features of an acute confusional state.

Other symptoms include hallucinations, particularly visual hallucinations, dysphasia and perseveration, disconnected thinking; anxiety, sometimes amounting to frank terror, can also be present, particularly in delirium tremens (see below).

An acute confusional state can be caused by a wide variety of conditions; anything which interferes with brain function can bring it about. However, the clinical picture is largely the same whatever the pathogenesis; it is determined not so much by the primary cause as by: (i) the intensity and duration of the cerebral disturbance; (ii) the environmental stimuli present during the cerebral disturbance; (iii) the previous personality and experience of the patient.

Treatment must first be directed towards the underlying cause, and in many cases this will be sufficient to improve the psychological state. When rapid improvement of the basic disturbance is not possible, and the behaviour of the patient remains disturbed, then additional treatment specifically directed towards improving the mental state is usually indicated. In most cases cautious medication with chlorpromazine (Largactil, Thorazine) (see chapter 6) will suffice. As cerebral function is already impaired, and a lowered blood pressure accompanies many of the conditions producing an acute confusional state, it is essential to start treatment with a relatively small dose: 25–50 mg either orally or intramuscularly. Haloperidol (Haldol, Serenace) 2–5 mg is a useful alternative drug which is less prone to cause hypotension. If this does not produce the desired effect, and provided that there has been no worsening of the patient's clinical condition, the drug can be given subsequently in a larger dose: 50–100 mg. Occasionally it may be necessary to exceed 150 mg but this must be done with great care as most patients with an acute confusional state are already physically ill; adding what amounts to yet another toxic substance may well not improve matters overall.

In patients with liver failure the impaired detoxication of many anxiolytic sedatives and narcotics leads to an exaggeration and prolongation of their pharmacological effects; thus great caution must be exercised.

Delirium tremens

In contrast to other toxic confusional states, delirium tremens arises as a result of withdrawal of a drug (alcohol) rather than its administration. In order to reduce these withdrawal symptoms, which are very alarming and can even prove fatal, it is advisable to prescribe one of the benzodiazepine group of drugs, or chlormethiazole. Relatively large doses, given either orally or systemically, are usually required for adequate sedation: chlordiazepoxide (Librium) 25–50 mg, diazepam (Valium) 20–40 mg or chlormethiazole (Heminevrin) 1.5–2 g are probably the drugs of choice. In severe cases larger doses of these drugs may be required. When oral administration is not possible either chlormethiazole or chlordiazepoxide can be given by intravenous infusion.

A generally applicable treatment programme for the majority of cases of delirium tremens is chlormethiazole 6 g daily in divided doses for two days; 4 g daily for the next two days; 2 g daily for a further two days; 1 g daily for a final two days. It is necessary to tail off the drug as quickly as this in order to avoid the very real possibility of a secondary dependence to chlormethiazole developing. A further complication can arise in patients with respiratory disease as chlormethiazole has a tendency to increase secretions within the respiratory tract.

Patients with severe delirium tremens can rapidly become severely dehydrated. Should this happen appropriate measures must be taken urgently to correct their fluid and electrolyte balance; such measures may be life-saving. Finally, chronic alcoholism is often accompanied by a relative deficiency of thiamine and other B vitamins. Because of this, large doses of B vitamins are usually given systemically to patients with delirium tremens (see also chapter 10).

Dementia

Dementia, a condition characterised by a waning of intellectual powers, impairment of memory (particularly the retention of new information), emotional lability, a coarsening of the personality together with increasing disinterest in personal appearance and hygiene, comes about as a result of degeneration or destruction of the cerebral cortex. This may be caused by a variety of conditions, including the degenerative diseases (Huntington's chorea, Pick's

203

disease, Alzheimer's disease), trauma, toxic substances (lead and mercury), metabolic disturbance (prolonged hypoglycaemia, myxoedema), pernicious anaemia, infections (particularly syphilis), and neoplasms. However, more common than any of the above are cerebral arteriosclerosis and primary degeneration of the Alzheimer type, both occurring much more frequently in the elderly. Recent surveys have revealed that of those aged sixty-five or over about 5 per cent are suffering from frank dementia and another 5 per cent are suffering from a milder form. The great majority in both categories are living in the community, institutional care being provided for relatively few. Most have dementia of the Alzheimer type (senile dementia); the remainder are suffering from cerebral degeneration secondary to artiosclerosis, giving rise to multi-infarct dementia. Before considering any drug treatment (see below) close attention should always be paid to providing adequate social and personal support.

Senile dementia of the Alzheimer type

In many respects senile dementia of the Alzheimer type can be seen as a gross exaggeration of the normal aging process, although whether the two differ qualitatively as well as quantitatively is an open question. Although normal aging is associated with the appearance of Alzheimer plaques (argentophil plaques) in the cerebral cortex, in senile dementia there are many more such plaques, and the greater the number of plaques the more severe the dementia. In contrast to multi-infarct dementia, the course is continuous and there are few, if any, focal neurological signs. There may be a family history of senile dementia, and it is this genetic predisposition which leads some authorities to consider that senile dementia is distinct from normal aging. Within the cerebral cortex hippocampus and the amygdala the levels of choline acetyl-transferase and acetylcholinesterase have been found to be reduced. These enzymes are involved in the metabolism of the neurotransmitter acetylcholine and it might be that the patho-genesis of this condition is related to a failure in the cholinergic system in the brain. These findings have stimulated attempts to overcome the failure of the cholinergic system by treating patients with the acetyl choline precursors choline or lecithin in order to promote synthesis of acetylcholine. Piracetam, which stimulates the release of acetylcholine, has also been tried. Another tactic has been to prevent the breakdown of already existing acetylcholine within the brain using the cholinesterase inhibitor physostigmine. Thus far such therapeutic approaches have proved to be disappointingly inconsistent. This might be due to involvement of other neurotransmitter systems in the pathogenesis of the illness. Less elderly patients (i.e. those developing symptoms of dementia before the age of 80) show a more widespread neurochemical abnormality than the older group (aged 80 and above). Whereas in the oldest patients the major neurochemical disturbance is confined to the cholinergic system in the temporal lobe and hippocampus, in the less old there are, in addition to cholinergic deficits which in this group involve the frontal cortex, changes in neurone systems involving noradrenaline, gamma-amino butyric acid and somato-statin. These latter changes are quite distinct from those occurring in normal aging.

Neurophysiologically there is often a slowing in the frequency and in the amount of the alpha rhythm in the EEG. There is also a slowing of conduction time in peripheral nerves, as well as a significant increase in latency in the EEG-recorded somatosensory evoked response. These findings suggest that the basic disturbance in senile dementia may be a generalised slowing of conduction within the nervous system.

There is no known treatment which effectively reverses or even halts the underlying pathological process. Controlled trials of a wide variety of substances including folic acid, androgenic hormones and procaine hydrochloride (substance 'H') have shown them all to be quite ineffective. The same strictures apply to the vasodilator drugs which have proven as ineffective in the treatment of senile dementia as in multi-infarct dementia (see below).

The only drug which has shown any therapeutic promise in this condition is the dihydrogenated ergot alkaloid dihydroergotoxine (Hydergine). It is administered orally or sublingually at an initial dose of 1 mg three times daily. Mild nausea is a frequently reported side effect. Most benefit is seen in cases exhibiting early symptoms of dementia, and even here the effect is likely to be only modest; no improvement can be expected in severely demented patients. Many patients, particularly in the later stages of the disease, exhibit disturbed behaviour both during the day and in the night. The most suitable drug for day-time control is thioridazine (Mellaril) in a dose of 25–100 mg given up to three times daily. While extrapyramidal symptoms are less likely with this drug than

205

with other phenothiazine compounds, there is a risk of retrolental fibroplasia and of retinitis if a daily dosage of 600 mg is continued for more than a few months. A suitable alternative drug is haloperidol 0.5–6 mg daily, but here the risk of extrapyramidal reactions is greater; should these occur an antiparkinsonian agent may be required in addition (see chapter 6).

For night sedation chloral hydrate given as syrup or as dichloralphenazone (Welldorm) 650–1300 mg is suitable (see chapter 11). Barbiturates should be avoided. Other possible alternatives include chlormethiazole (Heminevrin) and a benzodiazepine drug such as temazepam (Euhypnos, Normison) 10 mg or 0.5–1.0 g in tablet form; in many cases the syrup form may prove more acceptable; up to 20 mg may be required.

Multi-infarct dementia

Dementia due to cerebral vascular disease tends to run a fluctuating course. In addition, there are usually focal neurological signs together with a raised blood pressure. Post-mortem studies reveal widespread areas of cerebral softening. The greater the degree of intellectual impairment present the greater the total area of cerebral softening found. Unfortunately, treatment of established arteriosclerosis is largely unavailing; certainly by the time dementia has occurred no measures designed to alter such factors as the general blood pressure level are likely to do much good. However, some claims have been made for cyclandelate (Cyclospasmol), isoxsuprine (Duvadilan) and dihydroergotoxine (Hydergine) which appear to increase cerebral blood flow; improvement in intellectual capacity and memory has been reported after a few months continuous treatment with cyclandelate 400 mg four times daily. Unfortunately, there appeared to be no correlation between the degree of improvement in cerebral circulation observed with radio-circulograms and the level of improvement in psychometric test scores. Furthermore, the ward nursing staff failed to note any greater improvement in the patients given cyclandelate as compared to those given placebo. A more recently introduced compound naftidrofuryl (Praxiline) has proved superior to placebo in controlled trials. However, until more comprehensive studies have been completed the place of these drugs in the treatment of arteriosclerotic dementia must remain uncertain, and their routine use in the elderly showing mental impairment has not yet been justified. Treatment of associated disturbed behaviour is as for senile dementia (see above).

Dysmnesic syndrome (Korsakoff's psychosis)

Although profound memory disturbance occurs in acute confusional states and in dementia, it is but a part, albeit an important part, of a much wider disturbance of psychological function. The term 'dysmnesic syndrome' refers to those cases in which there is a considerable impairment in the cerebral mechanism underlying the process of remembering without any clouding of consciousness (as in acute confusional state) and without any general deterioration in intellect (as in dementia). Most commonly the dysmnesic syndrome follows Wernicke's encephalopathy, itself a consequence of chronic alcoholism. When this happens the condition is synonymous with Korsakoff's psychosis; there are, however, other possible causes including encephalitis, trauma, tumours of the third ventricle and carbon monoxide poisoning.

In the dysmnesic syndrome the major defect is in the retention of new information. Patients can recognise new information perfectly well, and are able to repeat it for a period of a few minutes afterwards. Yet, within a relatively short time they have no recollection of it whatsoever. The consolidation of new information into the memory store is completely blocked. Although the biochemical and physiological basis for memory is as yet ill-understood, there is greater knowledge regarding the anatomy. Bilateral lesions limited either to the mammillary bodies (as in Korsakoff's psychosis) or to the hippocampus are sufficient to produce the full clinical picture of the dysmnesic syndrome.

The inability to retain new information results in patients becoming disoriented in time and space so that they may not remember such things as the day of the month or where they are. Many patients realise their deficiencies in this regard and when pressed will invent answers to fill the gaps (confabulation). Such confabulation is, however, not an essential component of the syndrome. It has been suggested that long-term memory storage is associated with subtle alterations of chemical substances within the brain. As ribose nucleic acid (RNA) was thought to be involved, attempts have been made to provide extra RNA to patients with the dysmnesic syndrome in the hope of improving their capacity to remember. Thus far the results of such attempts have been

207

disappointing, and any improvement noted did not appear to be permanent. While administration of thiamine is unlikely to affect any marked change in memory it should be given a trial either parenterally or orally, particularly in the early stages (see chapter 10).

Huntington's chorea

This is a hereditary condition, transmitted by an autosomal dominant gene with each child of an affected patient standing a 50:50 chance of developing the disease. As it does not normally come before the third or fourth decade, there is a considerable risk that a genetically predisposed individuals will have fathered or borne children before knowing they were going to get it themselves. Typically choreiform movements precede the onset of a progressive dementia.

Histologically, there is marked atrophy of the caudate nucleus and putamen. Recent neurochemical studies have indicated that the neurotransmitter gamma-aminobutyric acid (GABA) and its biosynthetic enzyme, glutamic acid decarboxylase, are significantly reduced in the globus pallidus, the substantia nigra, the caudate nucleus and the putamen. The finding that GABA receptors are intact would imply that treatment with GABA-mimetic drugs might prove useful in modifying the choreiform movements, although they would not be likely to influence the course of the progressive dementia. Unfortunately, treatment with sodium valproate (Epilim), a compound found to elevate brain GABA in animals by inhibiting glutamate transaminases, has thus far proved disappointing. The loss of the inhibiting action by GABA on dopaminergic (DA) neurones (see chapter 2) may result in an increased DA effect. In keeping with this, phenothiazine compounds, which block DA receptors, currently afford the best available treatment. Thioridazine (Melleril) 50–150 mg or tetrabenazine (Nitoman) 25 mg two or three times daily are probably the most generally useful drugs in the management of Huntington's chorea.

Gilles de la Tourette syndrome

This is an uncommon, genetically determined disorder coming on in childhood. It is characterised by repetitive muscular tics involving the facial muscles most commonly although many other muscle groups may be affected, plus involuntary vocalisations containing a high frequency of obscenities (coprolalia).

An abnormality of the dopaminergic system in the basal ganglia has been implicated in the pathogenesis of the condition. There is a lowering of the dopamine (DA) metabolite, homovanillac acid in the CSF of patients compared to control subjects, and symptoms are exacerbated by the DA agonists l-dopa, bromocriptine and amphetamine, while DA receptor blocking drugs such as haloperidol and pimozide (see chapter 6) have been found to lessen tic frequency and vocalisations. It appears that the abnormality affects particularly D_2 receptors (see chapter 2) as the specific D_2 receptor blocking drug piguindone is at least as effective as haloperidol.

Another drug which has been tried is clonidine, an alpha-2 adrenergic agonist (see chapter 2). This appears to influence the associated behaviour disturbance more than the involuntary movement.

Suggestions for further reading

BIRD, E. D., and IVERSEN, L. L., 'Neurochemical findings in Huntington's chorea', in *Essays in Neurochemistry and Neuropharmacology*, vol. 1, ed. M. B. H. Youdim, W. Lovenberg, D. F. Sharman and J. R. Lagnado, John Wiley, Chichester, 1977.

CORSELLIS, J. A. N., 'The pathology of dementia', in *Contemporary Psychiatry*, ed. T. Silverstone and B. Barraclough, *British Journal of Psychiatry* Special Publication, no. 9, 1975.

CRAMOND, W. A., 'Organic Psychosis', *British Medical Journal*, vol. 4, 1968, pp. 497–500.

DAVIES, P., and MALONEY, A. J. F., 'Selective loss of central cholinergic neurones in Alzheimer's disease', *Lancet*, vol. 2, 1976, p. 1403.

DRUG AND THERAPEUTICS BULLETIN, 'Drugs for dementia', vol. 13, 1975, pp. 85–7.

HIER, D. B., and CAPLAN, L. R., 'Drugs for senile dementia', *Drugs*, vol. 20, 1980, pp. 74–80.

LAWDEN, M., 'Gilles de la Tourette syndrome: a review', *Journal of the Royal Society of Medicine*, vol. 79, 1986, pp. 282–8.

LEVY, R., 'The neurophysiology of dementia', in *Contemporary Psychiatry*, ed. T. Silverstone and B. Barraclough, *British Journal of Psychiatry* Special Publication no. 9, 1975.

LISHMAN, W. A., *Organic Psychiatry*, Blackwell, Oxford, 1978.

MOLIS, R. C., DAVIS, B. M., JOHNS, C. A., MATHE, A. A., GREENWALD, B. S.,

HORVATH, T. B., and DAVIS, K. L., 'Oral physostigmine treatment of patients with Alzheimer's disease', *American Journal of Psychiatry*, vol. 142, 1985, pp. 28–33.

ROSSOR, M. N., IVERSEN, L. L., REYNOLDS, G. P., MOUNTJOY, C. Q., and ROTH, M., 'Neurochemical characteristics of early and late onset types of Alzheimer's disease', *British Medical Journal*, vol. 288, 1984, pp. 961–4.

YESAVAGE, J. A., TINKELBERG, J. R., HOLLISTER, L. E., and BERGER, P. A., 'Vasodilators in senile dementias', *Archives of General Psychiatry*, vol. 36, 1979, pp. 220–4.

Substance abuse, personality disorders and sexual deviance 10

Alcohol dependence

Someone suffering from alcohol dependence (alcoholism) may be defined as an individual who causes problems for himself, or creates difficulties for others, by reason of excessive drinking. Although the detailed pattern of alcohol consumption may vary from patient to patient, no resolution of these problems and difficulties is likely to take place without a drastic overall reduction of alcohol intake. Alcoholism is extremely prevalent in most Western societies; in the UK the estimated total number is over half a million. The situation in the USA is even worse; there, according to some authorities, about five million can be described as alcoholics, at an annual cost to the community of over a billion dollars.

The exact place of drug treatment in this condition has not yet been clearly established. It would appear to be of considerable benefit in the withdrawal phase, of probable benefit in some patients as a deterrent to further drinking, and of possible benefit in reducing the desire for alcohol in abstinent ex-alcoholics.

Withdrawal symptoms

When someone who has been regularly consuming large quantities of alcohol suddenly stops drinking altogether, he may well experience withdrawal symptoms, which are a consequence of physical dependence on the drug. These can vary from mild nausea, tremulousness, headaches and general malaise to frank delirium tremens.

When mild, these symptoms usually require little more than a period of rest, together with one of the benzodiazepine drugs, either chlordiazepoxide (Librium) 30–75 mg or diazepam (Valium) 15–30 mg three times daily; an equally effective alternative is chlormethiazole (Heminevrin) 1–1.5 mg two or three times daily. When the risk of convulsions is high the anticonvulsant carbamazepine (Tregretol) 200 mg twice daily may be preferred (see chapter 7).

In contrast, the serious condition of frank delirium tremens calls for much more vigorous treatment. Clinical management includes the recognition and treatment of any concurrent medical condition, and the maintenance of an adequate fluid balance. In some cases emergency measures to counter profound hypothermia or severe hypotension may be necessary; in any case a regular watch must be maintained on temperature, pulse and blood pressure.

Treatment of the delirium itself is with larger doses of chlordiazepoxide or diazepam, or with chlormethiazole, either orally or by intravenous infusion (for details of treatment see chapter 9).

As many patients who have reached this stage in their condition have long-standing nutritional deficiencies, it is not unreasonable to administer large doses of high-potency vitamins systemically, although it should be appreciated that there is no evidence to suggest that vitamins are in any way a specific remedy for delirium tremens.

Deterrence from further drinking

Quite by chance, two doctors who had been taking disulfiram (Antabuse) in the course of an investigation into its possible use as an antihelminthic, experienced a series of extremely unpleasant physical reactions after attending a cocktail party. They were quick to conclude that the drug they had been taking had interfered with their metabolism of alcohol thus producing a toxic reaction; disulfiram by itself had produced no such ill-effects. As a result of this observation, disulfiram was given to selected alcoholics, who although they wished to stop drinking lacked the necessary resolve to persevere. They knew that if they drank after taking disulfiram they would experience marked ill-effects, due to the presence of acetaldehyde in their circulation. The serum acetaldehyde level rises because disulfiram competes with the acetaldehyde formed from the metabolism of alcohol for the enzyme aldehyde-NAD-oxidoreductase (ALDH). The competitive inhibition of this enzyme causes the blood level of acetaldehyde to rise, producing a syndrome called the disulfiram–ethanol reaction (DER) which is characterised by widespread vasodilation (causing a violent throbbing sensation), vomiting, chest pain and dyspnoea. In addition there is a pronounced fall in blood pressure, leading to vertigo, blurred vision, and eventual collapse. In addition to causing the plasma level of acetaldehyde to rise, disulfiram, through its metabolite diethyldithiocarbamate, inhibits the enzyme dopamine-β-hydroxylase which converts dopamine (DA) to noradrenaline (NA) (see chapter 2). This results in a relative rise in DA and fall in NA. The DER can be viewed as being due to the combined effects of an accumulation of acetaldehyde plus a deficiency of NA on the myocardium and on the arterioles. The rationale behind such treatment is the hope that, in order to avoid the acetaldehyde syndrome, an alcoholic will desist from drinking once he has taken his daily disulfiram. As long as he continues to take it the potential effect will remain; however, if the patient stops taking his daily disulfiram, within a week all its effects will have worn off, and he will feel no symptoms of the acetaldehyde syndrome no matter how much he may drink. Unfortunately, this approach helps only that relatively small proportion of alcoholics whose resolve is sufficient to ensure regular administration of their disulfiram, but who without their deterrent might weaken during the course of the day. Some intrepid patients even 'drink through' their acetaldehyde reaction, potentially a highly dangerous procedure. Because of this possibility patients must be very carefully selected before being placed on a disulfiram treatment programme. It should not be used in the elderly or in those with pre-existing cardiovascular disease, pronounced liver damage, epilepsy, asthma or diabetes.

It is no longer considered necessary to submit every patient to a preliminary test with disulfiram, or citrated calcium carbimide (see below), plus alcohol; such a procedure carries some risk. After an initial loading dose, a maintenance dose of disulfiram of one tablet containing 0.2 g daily is sufficient for most patients. Some patients, however, particularly those who relapse while taking disulfiram, may require a somewhat larger dose.

Although disulfiram by itself was originally thought to be without ill-effect, experience has revealed that depression, malaise, bad breath (due to a garlic-like flavour), impotence, gastro-intestinal symptoms, and occasionally peripheral neuropathy may be produced by the drug, particularly at a dose level higher than 0.5 g per day; drowsiness is common. Cases of a frank psychosis closely resembling schizophrenia have been reported. As in other drug-related schizophreniform psychoses (see chapter 6) this is possibly due to a rise in intracerebral DA which in this instance results from dopamine-beta-hydroxylase inhibition. Because of these effects many patients are reluctant to persist in taking disulfiram for a sufficient length of time, and consequently relapse. There is also evidence that it may influence the anticoagulant activity of warfarin and interfere with prothrombin control.

As an alternative, a citrated calcium carbimide (Abstem, Temposil) which produces similar effects in combination with alcohol has the advantage of being much more rapidly metabolised and thus less likely to produce unwanted side effects. This is also due to the fact that calcium carbimide is a reversible inhibitor of ALDH in contrast to disulfiram which is an irreversible inhibitor. Nor does calcium carbimide inhibit dopamine-beta-hydroxylase. The required dose is 50–100 mg per day.

While long-term drug therapy of the deterrent type may help some alcoholics, the great majority require repeated or continuous psychological and social support; the part which drugs can play in the long-term management of this condition is at present very limited.

Finally, it should not be forgotten that some individuals are what might be considered symptomatic drinkers; that is, they drink excessively only when they become depressed as part of an affective disorder or develop symptoms of acute anxiety. In every case of alcoholism an attempt should be made to recognise any such precipitating factors; if present they should be treated promptly. Alleviation of any underlying depression (see chapter 7) or anxiety state (see chapter 8) will often reduce the patient's need to consume the alcohol which he had previously required for relief of his psychological distress.

Treatment of neurological complications

1   Wernicke's syndrome of ataxia, diplopia and confusion requires urgent treatment with replacement thiamine. Parenteral administration of 50 mg thiamine daily is recommended until the clinical state has improved sufficiently, when oral administration can be substituted.

2   The dysmnesic syndrome (Korsakoff's psychosis) (see chapter 9), which may occur in long-standing alcoholism, is less responsive

to thiamine replacement, but its onset may be prevented by early and adequate thiamine replacement whenever there is evidence of diplopia or of cerebellar signs.

3   Alcoholic polyneuropathy should be treated with a combination of thiamine, pantothenic acid, nicotinic acid and pyridoxine, as deficiencies of all these substances are thought to play a part in the pathogenesis of the neuropathy. Treatment should continue for several months as resolution of symptoms can be slow.

Drug dependence (substance abuse)

Psychological and, in many instances, physiological dependence on drugs is an ever-increasing problem in our society, particularly among the young. Drug dependence is by no means limited to illegal drugs such as heroin, cocaine, cannabis and amphetamine. Numerically there is a much larger problem of dependence on commonly prescribed preparations such as the benzodiazepines (see chapter 8) and a variety of analgesic preparations. Furthermore it should be recognised that individuals who abuse this type of drug are likely to be taking a variety of other drugs as well according to fashion, availability and personal preference.

Drug dependence has been defined by the World Health Organisation as:

A state, psychic and sometimes also physical, resulting from the interaction between a living organism and a drug characterised by behavioural and other responses that always include a compulsion to take the drug on a continuous or periodic basis in order to experience its psychic effects and sometimes to avoid the discomfort of its absence. Tolerance may or may not be present. A person may be dependent on more than one drug.

Some further WHO definitions of the terms used are as follows:

Tolerance: 'the phenomenon of dose increase to maintain the drug effect'.
Physical dependence: 'an adaptive state that manifests itself by intense physical disturbances when the administration of the drug is suspended or when its action is affected by the administration of a specific antagonist'.

215

Psychological dependence: 'a condition in which a drug produces a feeling of satisfaction and a psychic drive that require periodic or continuous administration of the drug to produce pleasure or to avoid discomfort'.

Drugs likely to lead to dependence all have in common the property of producing a rapid change of mood, or reduction of tension, followed by a feeling of 'let-down', which in turn can only be relieved by taking more of the drug.

Clinical features of dependence vary with the drug in question, and can best be considered in relation to the groups of compounds causing dependence, namely: (1) opiate derivatives; (2) antianxiety and hypnotic drugs; (3) stimulant drugs; (4) cannabis and other hallucinogenic drugs; (5) solvents.

While the pattern of dependence may vary with the drug, the personalities of the individuals who become dependent tend to be similar. The most frequent type of personality observed in a patient presenting with drug dependence can broadly be described as 'inadequate'; he is often someone who has difficulty in coping with the normal frustrations of life. Such a person often seeks immediate gratification, finding any delay intolerable, with a consequent tendency to impulsive and ill-considered behaviour. There are, of course, many people with similar characteristics who are not drug-dependent, but the addict has found or selected a particular way, namely the use of centrally acting drugs, of coping with his emotional problems and gratifying his psychological needs. It should be noted that not all addicts show this characteristic personality structure, and social and environmental factors play a large part in determining the occurrence and the pattern of drug abuse and drug dependence.

1 *Dependence on opiate derivatives* The use and abuse of opiates dates from pre-history, but it was not considered a social problem until the eighteenth century. At that time the East India Company exploited the addictive properties of opium commercially, and this in turn led to the opium wars in the next century. Following the introduction of injectable morphine into military medicine during the American Civil War, a number of soldiers became dependent, a condition referred to at the time as the 'soldier's disease'. Heroin, originally produced as a non-addictive alternative to morphine, proved itself an even greater menace and most opiate addicts in

Western society now take heroin, often intravenously. In the 1950s and 1960s most addicts dependent on heroin were prescribed the drug legally by doctors. After the change in the law, in the UK at least the pattern of heroin dependence has changed dramatically with far more young 'non-therapeutic' addicts being introduced to drug taking by their friends. The addict's first experience of heroin often occurs when the friend, who may already be dependent, encourages the other to try it. People starting on heroin generally begin by sniffing the powder ('snorting'); this is followed by heating the powder and inhaling the vapour ('chasing the dragon'). The user may go on to self-injection ('fixing'), which when intravenous is called 'mainlining'. The first experience of heroin is frequently accompanied by nausea, but the euphoriant effect leads the subject to try again. The first few injections may be subcutaneous but these soon give way to intravenous injections ('mainlining') which gives a more immediate sensation ('buzz'). At first, heroin injections will be limited to occasional weekend use, but self-injection soon becomes more frequent until, within a matter of months, the addict is no longer injecting heroin for positive pleasure; he is desperately trying to avoid the unpleasant effects accompanying withdrawal. These include shivering with pilo-erection (hence the term 'cold-turkey'), watering of the eyes and running nose, abdominal cramp followed by vomiting and diarrhoea. Individuals vary considerably in the intensity with which such symptoms are experienced.

Perhaps the most disturbing aspect of heroin dependence is the high mortality of young, previously healthy, adults and adolescents. The mortality rate is twenty times that of non-addicts, and is due partly to secondary infection accompanying intravenous injections without sterile precautions, rather than to the direct action of the drug itself, although in some cases death follows an accidental overdose particularly when tolerance has waned following a period of abstinence. Another significant cause of death among this group is overdosage of other drugs taken in conjunction with, or as a substitute for, heroin.

Dependence on a number of opiate-related drugs can also occur. These include methadone (Physeptone) (it is used as a replacement for heroin in some treatment programmes, see below); dihydro-codeine (the acute constituent of the proprietary preparation DF 118); dextromoramide (Palfium); dextropropoxyphene, an analgesic contained in the proprietary preparation Distalgesic;

pentazocine (Fortral), which although an opiate partial agonist, has led to dependence. Buprenorphine (Temgesic), which has a mixed agonist and antagonist effect on opioid receptors, is also subject to abuse.

Recently a number of synthetic analogues of the opiate analgesics ('designer drugs') have been introduced in an attempt to circumvent the laws regarding existing products.

Opiates are readily absorbed from the gastrointestinal tract, through the nasal mucosa and from the lungs, but the subjective effects are experienced with more immediacy when the drugs are injected intravenously. This is why most addicts self-administer their drugs by intravenous injection with the consequent risk of infection.

Marked tolerance to opiate drugs occurs with regular administration; amounts of over 2.5 g a day of heroin have been taken without serious consequences by hardened addicts, doses which would be fatal in non-tolerant subjects. As tolerance rapidly subsides during abstinence, as can occur in prison, there is a real risk for the addict of taking a fatal overdose on his release from prison if he immediately reverts to self-administering heroin in the same dosage he did before entering prison.

It is considered that tolerance, and also withdrawal symptoms (see below) are related to adaptive changes taking place at opiate receptors within the tissues rather than to any changes in metabolism (as, for example, occurs with barbiturates). A possible mechanism is that during chronic opiate administration the inhibition of certain neurotransmitter systems normally exercised by endogenous enkephalin substances is produced by the exogenous opiate. This leads to a reduction in the formation and release of enkephalins, and on withdrawal of the exogenous opiates there is not enough enkephalin available to exert the normal inhibitory control in the relevant neurotransmitter systems. Whatever the mechanism of withdrawal symptoms, their severity is to a large degree determined by psychological factors; perhaps even more than by the duration of drug use or the doses taken.

Treatment is aimed at withdrawal and abstinence, either gradually on an out-patient basis, or rapidly in an in-patient unit. While in-patient withdrawal may be effective in the short term, longer-term management depends on a wide range of community services. Current practice is to place more emphasis on helping the addict to develop alternative coping strategies than on achieving abstinence as an end in itself.

2 *Dependence on antianxiety and sedative drugs*   (see chapter 8).

3 *Dependence on stimulant drugs (i) Amphetamine* Soon after the introduction of amphetamine in the early 1930s its stimulant and euphoriant properties became widely recognised, and amphetamine abuse created clinical and social problems within a very short time. By the 1950s the contents of amphetamine inhalers were being extracted on a large scale and ingested by young people in the UK, Scandinavia, the USA and Japan. When the availability of such inhalers was restricted, interest turned to amphetamine in tablet form, either alone or in combination with barbiturates (Drinamyl, 'Purple Hearts'). Illegally introduced amphetamine sulphate powder has now almost completely replaced amphetamine obtained from inhalers or other medicinal preparation.

Two quite distinct groups of people become dependent on amphetamine. First there are the otherwise relatively stable, often middle-aged women for whom amphetamine (and occasionally other stimulant anorectic drugs such as diethylpropion or phentermine) was prescribed to help them lose weight (see chapter 12); they seek repeated small doses of their stimulant anorectic to avoid the lethargy they experience when they are without the drug. The second group are much more emotionally unstable young adults or adolescents who take amphetamine to attain a state of euphoria and to ward off fatigue. As the effects wear off they experience a profound depression which can only be satisfactorily relieved by further amphetamine. Abuse in this group may lead to restlessness and irritability, resulting in unreasoning aggression towards others. On examination the pupils are dilated and there is a rapid pounding pulse. If amphetamine is taken over a long period a marked weight loss occurs.

Amphetamine psychosis can follow a number of large doses (50 to 100 mg) taken over a relatively short time. In this condition the patient is tormented by vivid auditory hallucinations and paranoid delusions. In some ways amphetamine psychosis resembles an acute schizophrenic episode but unlike schizophrenia the symptoms promptly wane when the drug is withheld.

Physical dependence to amphetamine probably occurs, in that a rebound increase in REM sleep is observed on sudden withdrawal. Nevertheless treatment is by simple withdrawal, although the possibility of a serious post-drug depressive state must be guarded against. Adequate social rehabilitation and psychological support will usually be required; and occasionally treatment with an antidepressant drug may be needed.

In the view of most medical authorities, amphetamines have little place in clinical practice, apart from narcolepsy and the hyperkinetic syndrome in children (see chapter 14).

(ii) Cocaine Cocaine, like amphetamine, is a central-nervous stimulant producing slight physical dependence. When taken in large doses it leads to a state of over-activity and excitement. Its use as a recreational drug has grown greatly in recent years. On occasions it can produce a most uncomfortable sensation in the skin reminiscent of insects crawling all over one's body (formication). Withdrawal symptoms when they occur tend to be mild; they consist of lassitude, drowsiness and depression. An even more intense stimulant effect can be obtained from free-base cocaine ('crack') which is becoming increasingly popular among illicit drug users.

4 *Dependence on drugs of the cannabis type* Probably no drug in recent times has been surrounded by more controversy and contention than cannabis, the mixture of substances obtained from Indian hemp. There are at least four pharmacologically active substances in the resin: (i) tetrahydrocannabinol (THC) which depresses acetylcholine release within the intestine; (ii) a second, closely related substance; (iii) a fat-soluble central-nervous depressant; (iv) a water-soluble atropine-like substance.

It is difficult to know exactly what the psychopharmacological effects of cannabis are, as the subjective experiences vary so much with the social conditions under which it is taken. Regular users report a hazy glow of contentment, accompanied by a sharpening of perception; in contrast, naive users often find that the effects, if any, are somewhat unpleasant. It produces little in the way of physiological effects apart from a rise in heart rate and a reddening of the conjunctiva. On psychological testing, cannabis was found to impair psychomotor performance in naive smokers but not in regular users.

High dosage can result in frank delirium and associated paranoid delusions followed by subsequent amnesia for the whole episode. Cannabis can lead to the exacerbation of a pre-existing schizophrenic illness.

5 *Dependence on hallucinogenic drugs* We have already noted how preparations, like mescaline, with hallucinogenic properties can

become incorporated into religious rites (see chapter 1). More recently, particularly since the development of remarkably potent synthetic hallucinogens like lysergic acid diethylamide (LSD), the ingestion of hallucinogens has spread to other societies, partly in the belief that they may be therapeutic, and partly in the hope that the perceptual experiences produced will widen artistic horizons.

The amounts of LSD required to produce psychological effects are minuscule, as little as one millionth of a gram per kilogram body weight being sufficient, and of this, only 1 per cent actually crosses the blood–brain barrier.

LSD produces autonomic, sensory and emotional effects, in that sequence, over the course of some twelve to twenty-four hours. The autonomic effects include gastrointestinal activity leading to vomiting and diarrhoea, pupil dilation, pilo-erection and tremor. Following these there is a dramatic alteration of visual perception which allows the subject to perceive the world in a quite extraordinarily novel way. It is this distortion of perception which so attracted to LSD certain intellectuals and artists who hoped to find a new stimulus to creativity through the drug. At the same time, or shortly afterwards, there is an awareness of a change in the quality of experience, which has been described in such terms as 'ecstatic', 'mystical', 'transcendental', but, as with many other drugs, these effects depend to a considerable degree on the social situation in which LSD is taken and the expectations of those taking it. Unfortunate sequelae to LSD can occur, particularly when the sensation of power and invulnerability displaces all caution. Under such conditions subjects may jump off buildings in the conviction that they cannot possibly come to harm. The LSD experience ('trip') may also give way to depression and consequent suicide.

Another drug which produces alteration of perception similar to LSD is psylocibin, the active ingredient of small mushrooms which are sometimes called 'magic' mushrooms. Yet another hallucino-genic substance is PCP (angel dust, phencyclidine), which is also taken by drug abusers.

Occasionally the alterations in perceptional experience are extremely frightening and unpleasant. Such a distressing experience is often referred to as a 'bad trip'. When this is particularly severe it may be necessary to administer a benzodiazepine drug for a short time, although in most cases repeated reassurance is sufficient. Another subjective phenomenon associated with hallu-

221

cinogenic drugs is the so-called 'flashback' in which the vivid perceptual changes first experienced while under the influence of LSD are re-experienced some time later without recourse to LSD.

Treatment of dependence on opiate drugs

While drug treatment plays a relatively minor part in the overall management of this condition (in the UK at least), it is of considerable use when dealing with withdrawal symptoms. Furthermore the substitution of oral methadone for intravenous diamorphine (heroin) has been widely advocated as the best way of coping with the situation, although the considerable disadvantages of substituting one narcotic for another are becoming more generally recognised. A third area in which drug treatment may be of some limited use is in the maintenance of abstinence, although continued social and psychological support is likely to be of more lasting value.

The management of withdrawal

In treatment centres in Great Britain drug withdrawal is usually a gradual process frequently undertaken under out-patient conditions. In these circumstances there is no appearance of the classical withdrawal symptoms: lacrimation, rhinorrthoea, yawning, pilo-erection and perspiration; proceeding to extreme restlessness, violent cramp-like pains, retching and vomiting, accompanied by tachycardia and raised blood pressure. However, when the drug is stopped abruptly, then the clinical picture of withdrawal, as just described, can be extremely distressing. Pharmacologically, the withdrawal symptoms can be terminated by administration of the drug to which the patient is addicted, but in most situations this is unlikely to be desirable, even if possible. A compound which has a similar pharmacological spectrum to heroin, such as methadone (Physeptone), can be given orally at a starting dose of 20 mg three times a day. Over the next few days the dose of methadone can be gradually reduced, with only minimal symptoms of withdrawal.

Another substance which has been reported as reducing the intensity of withdrawal symptoms is clonidine, an alpha-2-adrenergic receptor blocking drug. While clonidine reduces the autonomic accompaniment of withdrawal it has less effect on the subjective symptoms of discomfort.

Psychological factors play a large part in the manifestation of the withdrawal syndrome and a supportive reassuring approach can often itself greatly reduce the severity of the symptoms experienced.

Should a heroin addict appear in a doctor's surgery (office) or hospital casualty department (receiving room) showing clear physical withdrawal symptoms, he should be given methadone up to 20 mg orally and be watched while he takes it. Arrangements can then be made for him to attend an appropriate treatment centre within the next twenty-four hours.

A situation in which withdrawal symptoms may present a serious threat to life is in babies born to opiate-dependent mothers. The first signs may appear before delivery as foetal distress. Should this occur it is imperative to ensure that the mother receives sufficient opiate to counter the withdrawal symptoms in the foetus. After delivery the infant suffering from withdrawal symptoms usually presents with irritability and tremulousness, which may be accompanied by vomiting and diarrhoea, as well as yawning, sneezing, respiratory distress, excess mucous secretion and even convulsions. Prompt treatment with chlorpromazine, 1 mg/kg body weight every four hours, is essential. This dose may be reduced over the course of the next few days.

Drug substitution

Methadone substitution consists of administering a daily oral dose of methadone. The addict is frequently required to obtain his or her medication, which lasts him throughout the twenty-four-hour period, until he is due for his next dose. Recent studies have indicated that while withdrawal effects may be expected forty-eight hours after a methadone-free period, the effects of a derivative, l-α-acetylmethadone last longer, and administering acetylmethadone three times a week has been tried. Overall this approach has not worked. It has not reduced the number of heroin users, which is in fact rising steeply, nor has it helped addicts to reduce their consumptions of opioids. It can no longer be recommended.

Narcotic antagonists

Naloxone is a pure antagonist at opiate receptors, possessing no morphine-like activity of its own. Unlike partial-agonists, it reverses the actions of pentazocine and dextropropoxyphene and is the drug of choice for treating narcotic overdosage (see page 271). Naltrexone is another opioid receptor antagonist, but unlike naloxone it is effective when taken orally, and has a longer duration of action.

Nalorphine and cyclazocine are partial agonists, antagonising the effects of a narcotic drug, but producing effects that are similar to the narcotics, including miosis, vomiting and respiratory depression.

These substances have been used in the supportive treatment of abstinent ex-addicts in much the same way as disulfiram is used in alcoholism. The abstinent ex-addict is advised to take the agonist daily; he then knows that if he subsequently takes a narcotic he will experience withdrawal symptoms. Unfortunately, as with disulfiram in alcoholism, only a minority of the patients who are insufficiently motivated to maintain abstinence without any drug, are sufficiently conscientious in their self-medication to persist for long enough.

Personality disorder

The personality of an individual refers to that special combination of psychological traits which make him the particular person he is. It can be considered in much the same way as his physical constitution, which again is a unique amalgam of anatomical and physiological features.

While we can accurately measure such anatomical features (e.g. height), we are far less able to quantify the various personality traits. We are even uncertain about the number of traits involved. Nevertheless, personality theorists generally agree that the following are among the more important characteristics: neuroticism (anxiety-prone); obsessionality (meticulous); tendency to hysterical behaviour (self-centred, histrionic); psychopathy (antisocial); extraversion/introversion; reliability; independence.

All of us exhibit these traits to some degree; where we differ from one another is in the quantity, rather than the quality, by which they are expressed.

Personality traits can best be considered as continuous rather than discrete variables. For instance we are all somewhat prone to be anxious (i.e. neurotic); but, while some people are made anxious by the least disturbance in the environment, others hardly turn a hair, even in what to many would be a most alarming situation. The majority feel anxious in what would be generally accepted as anxiety-provoking circumstances such as examinations, job interviews and public performances. It is only when anxiety becomes extreme, or occurs under minimal stress, that treatment is indicated (see chapter 8).

Similarly, social conformity varies from one person to another: at one extreme is the self-sacrificing, saint-like person, at the other is the selfish, inconsiderate bully. It is this latter group to which the term *psychopath* or sociopath generally refers. Psychopathy is but one of the so-called personality disorders (character disorders). According to the *DSM III* classification, the following personality disorders can be distinguished:

Paranoid: Tendency to unwarranted suspiciousness and mistrust of others, with increased probability to take offence, in cold unemotional individuals.

Schizoid: Emotional coldness and aloofness, in socially isolated person.

Histrionic: Overly dramatic and self-centred behaviour, with shallow emotions.

Narcissistic: Self-important, with exaggerated appraisal of abilities which require repeated admiration.

Antisocial: Repeated delinquent behaviour, with no concern for the rights and feelings of others.

Borderline: Impulsive and unpredictable behaviour; forms unstable, but intense, personal relationships in a setting of affective instability.

Dependent: Allows others to assume responsibility and subordinates own needs. Self-deprecating.

Compulsive: Perfectionists; preoccupation with details, indecisive, excessively tidy.

Passive–aggressive: Resists demands for adequate performance by 'intentional' inefficiency or stubbornness.

It is only when the abnormality of personality causes actual suffering to the individual concerned, or to society in general, that the term 'disorder' is justified.

Unfortunately for most of these conditions treatment has relatively little to offer in terms of 'cure'. Indeed, the very concept of cure is misconceived in this group of patients; we might just as well speak of 'curing' someone with an IQ of 70. All we can do is to help the patient get along with the psychological constitution (personality and intelligence) he has. Certainly by the time adulthood is reached, there is little, if any, hope of significantly influencing personality; we cannot turn the chronic worrier into a devil-may-care sort of fellow, nor can we easily transfer the callous psychopath into a model citizen. We may, however, through a psychotherapeutic approach, allow the patient to appreciate how his (or her) personality tends to produce or exacerbate certain situations, and how he or she affects other people. In addition, newer behavioural techniques offer great promise in this direction.

As far as drug treatment is concerned, the possibilities are limited. It is with the borderline disorders that most progress has been made, and here it is unclear how far these are reflections of underlying illnesses rather than simply reflecting exaggerated personality traits. Clinical trials have shown low-dose adjunctive treatment with antipsychotic drugs (see chapter 6) to be superior to treatment with antidepressant drugs (see chapter 7) as well as to placebo, particularly in those patients expressing ideas of reference, experiencing delusions and with a high level of anxiety (that is, patients with a more schizophreniform spectrum of symptoms). For the remainder, drug treatment is unlikely to produce any significant benefit and indeed may make the situation worse.

Sexual deviations

Sexual deviation is more common among men than among women, and men are more likely to commit grave antisocial acts in order to gratify their sexual desires. While no pharmacological agent can by itself alter the direction of sexual desire, oestrogens will reduce its strength. Either stilboestrol 5–10 mg daily or ethinyl oestradiol 0.02–0.05 mg daily can be used. Common side effects include nausea and gynaecomastia. Such an approach should only be considered when the sexual deviation is causing considerable distress to the individual concerned or there is a real danger of antisocial acts being committed. It is obvious that the whole-hearted cooperation of the patient is necessary.

The antiandrogen compound, cyproterone acetate in a daily dose of 10–20 mg given under controlled conditions has been shown to reduce libido and to reduce the erectile response to erotic stimulation. This effect of cyproterone is accompanied by a reduction of plasma testosterone. The DA receptor blocking compound benperidol (Anquil), although having a slight but definite effect on libido in a dose of 1 mg daily, does not appear to affect plasma testosterone levels.

An altogether different approach to sexual deviation involves the attempt to desensitise the patient to any possible anxieties he may have regarding normal heterosexual intercourse. This is based on the belief that many sexual perversions arise because of difficulties, either real or imagined, with heterosexual intercourse; relieving these difficulties should remove the need for deviant behaviour.

Suggestions for further reading

CALDWELL, J., *Amphetamine and Related Stimulants*, CRC Press, Boca Raton, Fla., 1980.

EDWARDS, G., and GRANT, M., *Alcoholism: New Knowledge and New Responses*, Croom Helm, London, 1977.

EDWARDS, G., and LITTLE, J., *Pharmacological Treatments for Alcoholism*, Croom Helm, London, 1984.

GLATT, M., *A Guide to Addiction and its Treatment*, MTP, Lancaster, 1974.

GUNDERSON, J. G., 'Pharmacotherapy for patients with borderline personality disorder', *Archives of General Psychiatry*, vol. 43, 1986, pp. 698–700.

JASINSKI, D. R., JOHNSON, R. E., and KOCHER, T. R., 'Clonidine in morphine withdrawal', *Archives of General Psychiatry*, vol. 42, 1985, pp. 1063–6.

MADDEN, J. S., *A Guide to Alcohol and Drug Dependence*, Wright, Bristol, 1974 (2nd edn).

NAHAS, G. G., and PATON, W. D. M., *Marihuana: Biological Effects*, Pergamon, Oxford, 1979.

ROYAL COLLEGE OF PSYCHIATRISTS, *Alcohol and Alcoholism*, Tavistock, London, 1979.

WORLD HEALTH ORGANISATION, *Report of the Expert Committee on Drug Dependence: 20th Report*, World Health Organisation Technical Reports, Series No. 551, 1974.

Sleep disturbance

11

Nature of sleep

Although sleep is an activity which occupies about one third of our life, its nature is still poorly understood. The notion that sleep is a state analogous to suspended animation, a state of cellular inactivity, was exploded when electroencephalographic records taken during sleep showed persistent electrical activity, but of a different character from that seen in the waking state. Furthermore, experiments in which subjects have been woken at frequent intervals have suggested that some sort of mental activity can go on all through the night, but that it is almost entirely, if not completely, forgotten on waking.

The sleep of newborn babies tends to be regulated more by their feeding schedule than by the clock. After this early period of life, however, sleep, in common with other factors such as body temperature and diuretic activity, is governed by a 24-hour rhythm. This in turn probably depends on the effects of alteration of light and darkness on hypothalamic centres and the pineal which then influence hormonal activities in other parts of the body through the pituitary gland. Fast air travel across the world has emphasised the importance of our learnt diurnal sleep rhythm. Many travellers find that it takes them several days to adjust their sleeping habits when they make long intercontinental journeys.

Even if some mental activity continues during sleep, there is no doubt that a sleeping person is in a state of inertia, being unresponsive to outside events. Electroneurophysiological studies in animals have shown that the reticular formation in the brain stem is intimately concerned with the state of consciousness and responsiveness. When the reticular formation is destroyed, leaving intact the main sensory pathways to the cerebral cortex, animals are in a perpetual sleep, confirmed by the EEG, even though

228

sensory impulses from the periphery still reach the cortex. When, on the other hand, sensory tracts to the cortex are divided above their afferent branches to the reticular formation, the animals sleep at intervals, but may be awakened by a stimulus such as noise. They waken spontaneously and are fully active between their sleep periods. If consciousness implies an awareness of a recognised stimulus and the ability to respond to it, then this is not possible without a cerebral cortex, and these latter animals cannot be said to be conscious. Wakefulness, however, is not the same as consciousness and is possible without a cerebral cortex. It is primarily dependent on the functional integrity of the reticular system.

Electrical activity of the brain in normal sleep may be divided into two phases:

1 *Slow-wave sleep* is characterised by large-amplitude, low-frequency waves at one to three cycles per second in which sleep is profound ('slow-wave sleep', 'orthodox sleep'). Brief bursts of faster activity at about 12 cycles per second are generally mixed in with these slow waves and are known as 'sleep spindles'.

2 *Rapid eye movement sleep* occurs at intervals between periods of orthodox sleep, and consists of low-amplitude, high-frequency, 'saw-tooth' waves accompanied by rapid conjugate movements of the eyes ('activated sleep', 'dream sleep', 'paradoxical sleep', 'rapid eye movement – REM – sleep'). Respiration, heart rate and blood pressure are irregular and the penis may be erect during this phase. If subjects are wakened while their EEG record shows evidence of REM sleep activity, they usually report that they were dreaming vividly. This phase occupies in all about a quarter of the total night's sleep, recurring about five times during the night. When wakened during orthodox sleep, subjects are more likely to report 'thinking' without emphasis on imagery, action or emotion.

Electroneurophysiologists have further divided orthodox sleep into four stages. Stage 1 is the lightest phase in which subjects are most easily wakened. As sleep deepens the EEG waves become slower and larger, reaching a maximum in Stage 4 sleep, which appears the most intense and from which it is most difficult to rouse the subject. Stages 3 and 4 occur mainly in the early part of the night and are most apparent in subjects who have been deprived of sleep.

Pharmacological basis of the stages of sleep

The role of neurotransmitter substances in producing the various stages of sleep is still uncertain and the evidence conflicting. Non-specific reduction of brain 5–HT and noradrenaline levels in animals by reserpine reduces both orthodox and REM sleep. Parachlorophenylalanine, a selective inhibitor of 5–HT synthesis, markedly decreases REM sleep in man, and this effect is antagonised by administration of 5-hydroxytryptophan, a pre-cursor of 5–HT. Administration of ɪ-tryptophan, also a precursor of 5–HT, increases orthodox sleep but reduces REM sleep. An important influence of 5–HT on sleep appears, therefore, to be clear.

Monoamine oxidase inhibitors, such as tranylcypromine, which increase brain concentrations of 5–HT, noradrenaline and dopamine lead to a progressive reduction in REM sleep and increase in orthodox sleep both in man and experimental animals, but whether this depends on the increase of 5–HT alone or involves catecholamines is not clear. The effects on sleep of drugs such as amphetamine and levodopa which selectively influence nor-adrenaline and dopamine synthesis or activity are controversial. Alpha adrenoceptors are believed to play an important role in the control of wakefulness and paradoxical sleep, and the involvement of beta adrenoceptors is indicated by the common experience that beta-receptor blocking drugs can markedly interfere with normal sleep and increase dream activity.

GABA and some short-chain fatty acids induce sleep in animals when injected parenterally under suitable conditions. The hypnotic effects of benzodiazepines, mediated through stimulation of benzodiazepine receptors, probably involve enhancement of GABA activity (see page 187).

Prolonged hypnotic effects and hangover

An ideal hypnotic drug should not only induce sleep rapidly and predictably, and maintain sleep for a reasonable length of time without markedly influencing the ratio of orthodox to REM sleep, but it should also be free from prolonged central effects. Studies with earlier benzodiazepine hypnotics such as nitrazepam have shown impairment of behavioural and psychomotor tests more than 12 hours after administration even though the subjects considered themselves alert and even if they were allowed their usual intake of coffee or tea. These results are not surprising when it is considered that the elimination half-life of nitrazepam is in excess of 20 hours in most subjects. Although the newer generation of hypnotic drugs such as temazepam and triazolam produce very much less residual impairment of psychomotor performance (Table 12), it is important to warn patients prescribed them of the possibility of diminished efficiency on the following day, particularly in relation to driving and other skills.

Withdrawal of hypnotic drugs

Abrupt withdrawal of hypnotics may be followed by insomnia. This tends to occur during the first night or so after withdrawal with rapidly eliminated drugs, but with the more slowly excreted drugs the fall in plasma concentration is relatively slow and sleep disturbance is delayed or may not occur at all. Rebound insomnia is particularly likely to occur when relatively high doses have been prescribed for several weeks or months, and it is important that such doses should be reduced in step-wise fashion over several days before complete withdrawal.

Dependence on hypnotic drugs

Benzodiazepine dependence (see chapter 8) may follow their prescription as hypnotics for insomnia. The risk can be reduced by the use of low doses for only a short period of time, followed by step-wise reduction and withdrawal.

Treatment of insomnia

Difficulty in sleeping is an extremely common complaint, as witnessed by the vast numbers of various sorts of sleeping tablets prescribed. It is estimated that some 600 million tablets or capsules are taken annually in the UK while the consumption in the USA is ten times as great. Of increasing importance is the frequency with which overdosage from sedative drugs occurs. With these factors in mind it should hardly be necessary to emphasise how important it is to avoid overenthusiastic medication for what is, after all, a condition which itself carries no risk.

Before deciding on a course of treatment it is necessary to

231

determine the causes of the sleep disturbance. Basically these are of four types:

(i) Secondary to some other condition producing discomfort, adequate treatment of which is the obvious first approach.

(ii) Environmental change in working patterns, or rapid shift from one time-zone to another as occurs in long-distance air travel. Shift workers who have to adjust to sleeping during the day one week, only to revert to nocturnal sleeping the following week, may find it difficult to go to sleep for a night or two after changing shifts. Here, cautious and limited use of hypnotic preparation is not unreasonable. A similar approach can be used for those travellers who may take a little while to adjust their diurnal rhythm to their new surroundings.

Another common environmental cause is having to sleep in strange surroundings, particularly in hospital, where an unfamiliar bed, the general unease felt by most when in hospital, and the noise made by other patients, all combine to prevent a good night's sleep. This is, of course, well recognised by medical and nursing staff. Some may consider that it is rather too well recognised in that it has become almost standard practice to prescribe night-time sedation for all patients before it is known whether or not they require it. Such practice is potentially harmful as many former patients become chronically dependent on sleeping tablets as a direct result of having first been given them while in hospital.

(iii) Certain illnesses are characterised by sleep disturbance which is an integral part of the condition. The most common such condition seen in psychiatric practice is depressive illness (endogenous depression), where early morning wakening is frequent. Patients describe how, although they can go to sleep without too much trouble, they waken in the early hours of the morning and are unable to go to sleep again. Their depression is often particularly severe at this time and the risk of suicide consequently high.

Although hypnotic drugs may help to relieve the early morning wakening, treatment of the underlying depressive illness will obviously be the first step in management (see chapter 7).

(iv) By far the most common cause of sleeping difficulty is worry or emotional strain: mothers worried about their children, husbands concerned over their job, adolescents crossed in love. All can lie awake, tossing and turning, brooding over their problems.

Eventually they nearly always get off to sleep, but do not feel refreshed when they waken to face their problems again. In many such cases frank discussion of their fears and worries may itself relieve the tension sufficiently to render any pharmacological intervention unnecessary.

Before prescribing drugs, simple non-drug measures should be taken as appropriate. For example, exercise, controlled sleep curtailment, together with caffeine and alcohol restriction may be sufficient to restore sleep in mild cases of insomnia.

Choice of drug treatment

Although there is a bewildering array of hypnotic drugs, in practice the most widely used in the United Kingdom are the benzo-diazepines and the chloral hydrate derivatives. The use of barbiturate drugs has markedly decreased as they have fallen into disfavour because of their danger in overdose, their habit-forming potential, their tendency to cause confusion in the elderly and their liver enzyme inducing properties.

Benzodiazepines

The choice of a particular benzodiazepine should ideally depend upon the clinical problem, namely whether it is desired to shorten sleep onset when there is difficulty in falling asleep, to prolong the sleeping time, or to produce an anxiolytic effect during the following day if insomnia is accompanied by anxiety. In practice this is not always possible.

(i) Drugs to shorten sleep onset must have a consistent rapid rate of absorption followed by short elimination half-life. The benzo-diazepines lormetazepam, temazepam and triazolam have these properties and are therefore suitable for this indication.

(ii) Prolongation of sleep time without residual effects on the following day is difficult to achieve with the drugs currently available, although some under investigation, including brotizolam and zolpidem, may possess the necessary duration of action. Nitrazepam, flurazepam and flunitrazepam, although widely used for this purpose, usually produce residual effects on the following day, and accumulate on repeated administration.

233

(iii) An anxiolytic action during the day following its hypnotic effect is particularly useful with diazepam, clorazepate and oxazepam, although the long-acting drugs given in paragraph (ii) (above) could also be used.

One major advantage of benzodiazepines over the barbiturates is safety in overdosage. However, respiratory depression can occur and they should be avoided, or used with great care, in patients with chronic respiratory disease. Unlike barbiturates, benzodiazepines do not induce liver enzymes, and are therefore safe in combination with oral anticoagulants (see page 193).

Chloral hydrate

This is a relatively weak hypnotic which, when absorbed, is metabolised to trichlorethanol. Its main disadvantage is its unpleasant taste and it also has an unfortunate tendency to produce gastric irritation. It should therefore be taken well diluted with milk or olive oil.

Triclofos sodium elixir causes fewer gastrointestinal effects. The preparation dichloralphenazone (Welldorm), which is in tablet form, may be a more acceptable way of administering the same compound, being particularly useful in the elderly.

Other drugs

Some MARI antidepressant drugs, particularly amitriptyline, have marked sedative qualities, and may be of value if depression is suspected as a cause of sleep disturbance.

The sedative antihistamine drugs promethazine and trimeprazine are useful for occasional use, particularly in children.

Narcolepsy

In this condition, the pathogenesis of which remains obscure, patients are frequently overtaken by irresistible attacks of sleep from which they can be readily wakened. Attacks, which may occur several times in one day, are characteristically brought on in susceptible individuals by emotional arousal. Narcolepsy is probably the only condition in adults for which administration of amphetamine is justified. It can be given either as the racemic mixture amphethamine sulphate (Benzedrine) or as the dextrorotatory-isomer, dexamphetamine sulphate (Dexedrine), both in a dosage of 5–10 mg three or four times a day. Methylphenidate (Ritalin) 10–20 mg two to four times daily is an effective alternative. Milder degrees of narcolepsy may respond to caffeine, either given as tablets (100–300 mg), or taken in coffee.

Recent evidence suggests that the MAO-B inhibitor selegiline (pages 35, 154) is as effective in treatment of narcolepsy as amphetamine. However, as its metabolic derivatives include amphetamine and methamphetamine, its mechanism of action in this condition is not clear.

Table 12   *Hypnotics*

Approved name	Proprietary name	Recommended dose	Elimination half-life (hours)	Remarks
Short acting benzodiazepines				
lormetazepam	Loranet Noctamid	0.5–1.0 mg	10	Useful for inducing sleep but less appropriate for treatment of early awakening
temazepam	Euhypnos Normison	5–60 mg	6	"
triazolam	Halcion	0.125–0.25 mg	3	"
Longer acting benzodiazepines				
flunitrazepam	Rohypnol	0.5–2.0 mg	16	May cause residual effects and accumulate
flurazepam	Dalmane Paxane	15–30 mg	40 (active metabolite)	"
loprazolam	Dormonoct	1.0–2.0 mg	8	Absorption is slow and variable
nitrazepam	Mogadon Nitrados Noctased Remnos Somnite Surem Unisomnia	5–10 mg	30	May cause residual effects and accumulate

Table 12   *contd.*

Approved name	Proprietary name	Recommended dose	Elimination half-life (hours)	Remarks
Others				
chloral hydrate	Noctec	0.5–1.0 g	8 (metabolite)	Safe, particularly useful in the elderly; may cause gastrointestinal symptoms
dichloral-phenazone	Welldorm	1.3–1.95 g	8	Relatively weak, but useful in the elderly
promethazine	Phenergan	25–75 mg	8	Useful for occasional use in children
triclofos sodium		1–2 g	8	Similar to chloral hydrate but better tolerated
trimeprazine	Vallergan	3 mg/kg (children)	24	Useful for occasional use in children

Suggestions for further reading

ADAM, K., ADAMSON, L., BREZINOVA, V., HUNTER, W. M., and OSWALD, I., 'Nitrazepam: lastingly effective but trouble on withdrawal', *British Medical Journal*, vol. 1, 1976, pp. 1558–60.

BREIMER, D. D., and JOCHEMSEN, R., 'Pharmacokinetics of hypnotic drugs', in *Psychopharmacology of Sleep*, ed. D. Wheatley, Raven Press, New York, 1981, pp. 135–52.

COMMITTEE ON THE REVIEW OF MEDICINES, 'Systematic review of the benzodiazepines', *British Medical Journal*, vol. 280, 1980, pp. 910–12.

GAILLARD, J. M., 'Biochemical pharmacology of paradoxical sleep', *British Journal of Clinical Pharmacology*, vol. 16, 1983, pp. 2055–305.

NICHOLSON, A. N., 'Hypnotics: their place in therapeutics', *Drugs*, vol. 31, 1986, pp. 164–76.

OSWALD, I., FRENCH, C., ADAM, K., and GILHAM, J., 'Benzodiazepine hypnotics remain effective for 24 weeks', *British Medical Journal*, vol. 284, 1982, pp. 860–3.

PRIEST, R. G., PLETSCHER, A., and WARD, J., *Sleep Research*, MTP, Lancaster, 1979.

SCHUTZ, H., *Benzodiazepines: A Handbook*, Springer-Verlag, Berlin, 1982.

Disorders of appetite and body weight $\qquad$ 12

Regulation of food intake and body weight

In most people energy intake, in the form of food, is closely matched to the energy expended by exercise and metabolic needs; and body weight remains more or less constant. When energy intake exceeds expenditure, due either to an increased food consumption without a concomitant increase in energy expenditure, or to a reduced expenditure without a concomitant reduction in food intake, body weight will increase. In other words a positive energy balance leads to weight gain. Conversely, a negative energy balance leads to weight loss.

Many factors contribute to both sides of the energy balance equation. Food intake is determined by physiological mechanisms in the central nervous system and in the periphery (see below), by psychological cues such as the sight, smell and taste of food, by the overt desire to gain or lose weight, which itself is often largely socially determined, and by clinical conditions such as depressive illness which usually causes a profound loss of appetite and secondary reduction in food intake (see chapter 7). Drugs too can profoundly affect the desire to eat; for example, chlorpromazine frequently increases appetite and leads to a significant weight gain in patients receiving it for long-term management of chronic schizophrenia (see chapter 6); while other drugs such as amphetamine reduce appetite, and consequently lead to weight loss. To understand how such drugs might act we need to consider the physiological mechanisms underlying the regulation of food intake. Although in the following sections the various systems thought to be involved in the regulation of food intake are considered separately, it should be recognised that their actions within the body are closely integrated.

Central nervous system

Until recently it was assumed, on the basis of earlier experiments on laboratory animals, that the hypothalamus held pride of place in the regulation of food intake, with the lateral hypothalamus being responsible for initiating feeding behaviour (the so-called 'feeding centre') and the ventro-medial hypothalamus being responsible for stopping eating (the so-called 'satiety centre'). It is now realised that this 'dual-centre' theory is an oversimplification. The two areas of the hypothalamus concerned contain many fibres from neurones arising in the brain stem which themselves affect feeding behaviour in animals. For example the lateral hypo-thalamus is closely associated anatomically with the median forebrain bundle in which there are dopaminergic (DA) pathways coming from the substantia nigra and associated structures, and noradrenergic (NA) fibres arising from the locus coeruleus and other brain stem nuclei (see Figure 1, p. 12). Lesions made in the dopaminergic pathways outside the hypothalamus produce the syndrome of aphagia and adipsia which was previously thought to be characteristic only of lateral hypothalamic lesions. Furthermore neurones utilising 5-hydroxytryptamine (5–HT) arising in the median raphe nuclei are also thought to be involved in feeding. In addition, other pathways descending from higher centres can influence feeding. Thus the neural regulation of food intake is now recognised to be extremely complex, and we can no longer talk of a single 'feeding centre' or 'satiety centre', each acting reciprocally on the other. It is more likely that many neuronal systems closely interact and no simple neurochemical or neuroanatomical theory can fully explain the regulation of food intake. Nevertheless the hypothalamus does play a part over and above that of acting as a simple relay station. Certain neurones in the lateral hypothalamus of the monkey have been found to respond to the sight of food only when the animal is food deprived, thus the lateral hypothalamus may act as a form of gating mechanism allowing certain stimuli to initiate feeding behaviour in one condition (food deprivation) but not in another.

It may be that certain pathways, especially the DA pathways, are more concerned with the execution of feeding behaviour while others are responsible for triggering off the behaviour: if this were so lesions in the DA pathways would reduce food intake, not by reducing the desire to eat (i.e. hunger) but by impairing the ability of the animal to eat. The NA pathways on the other hand could be more concerned with initiating feeding through a hunger mechanism which may be linked to some sort of general reward system. Even here the situation is not straightforward, for lesions in the ventral NA system which produce a marked increase in food intake reminiscent of ventromedial hypothalamic lesions, are dependent for their effect on an intact pituitary gland; so there would appear to be endocrine interactions as well.

Peripheral mechanisms

1   *Blood sugar and insulin*   It has long been known that insulin, which sharply lowers blood sugar, leads to a pronounced increase in subjective hunger, a property which has at times been made use of in treatment (see below). Closer examination of the relationship of blood sugar and hunger has revealed that this increased hunger does not begin to be experienced until the blood sugar starts to rise. As a result it has been suggested that it is not the absolute level of blood sugar but the rate of utilisation which is important in this connection. When there is a lot of insulin available and glucose utilisation is high there is no increase in hunger; it is only when the rate of glucose utilisation falls, and there is a reduced arterio-venous glucose difference, that hunger occurs. This view, often referred to as the 'glucostatic theory' is compatible with the clinical observation that diabetic patients with high blood sugar levels but low glucose utilisation rates due to lack of insulin, and a consequently low arterio-venous glucose difference, often feel very hungry. It should be emphasised however that within the physiological range of blood sugar utilisation rates there is little relationship to hunger; it would appear that the glucostatic mechanism acts only in conditions of extreme food deprivation.

2   *Carbohydrate absorption*   The rate of absorption of carbohydrate from the gastrointestinal tract into the hepatic portal vein appears to influence feeding in animals. The monitoring of this carbo-hydrate absorption may take place through glucoreceptors in the liver and signalled to the brain via the vagus.

It is difficult to know how important this mechanism is in man; vagotomy for peptic ulcer is not usually followed by obvious changes in subjective hunger. On the other hand rapid transit of food into the small intestine and subsequent rapid absorption does produce a syndrome (the 'dumping' syndrome) in which anorexia is a component. In any case rapid absorption of glucose calls forth a sharp rise in insulin secretion which in turn may affect hunger either via the glucostatic mechanism discussed above, or perhaps by a direct action in the central nervous system.

3 *Gastrointestinal motility* Perhaps the earliest theory of hunger regulation was that of Cannon who attributed the sensation of hunger almost entirely to contractions of the empty stomach which caused so-called 'hunger pangs'. Subsequent work has tended to cast doubt on this mechanism as a dominant factor, although in certain normal subjects periods of fasting gastric motility, which occur every 40 to 120 minutes and which last for some 15–20 minutes on average, are associated with a detectable increase in hunger ratings (see chapter 4), conversely the disappearance of this gastric motility is accompanied by a fall in hunger ratings. Furthermore on direct questioning the majority of normal people recognise a gastrointestinal component to their hunger sensations, although it is by no means certain that this is related to fasting gastric motility. An alternative view suggests that it is the rate of gastric emptying after a meal which determines the onset of hunger for the next meal. In keeping with this is the finding in experimental animals that administration of cholecystokinin (CCK), which is normally released when food enters the duodenum, can cause an animal to stop eating.

4 *Temperature and metabolic rate* It has been suggested that we eat merely to keep warm. Certainly food intake increases in cold weather, and temperature regulation could therefore be a significant determinant of food intake. In Western society, however, the ambient temperature indoors is usually controlled to within very narrow limits by such devices as central heating and air conditioning, and when we go out into the cold weather we simply put on extra clothing, thereby literally insulating ourselves against the more extreme temperatures. It may nevertheless be the case that temperature has a bearing on food intake in certain circumstances.

Changes in metabolic rate certainly can affect food intake. It is a frequent clinical observation that patients suffering from hyperthyroidism with a consequent increase in metabolic rate, are voraciously hungry. In fact, significant loss of weight in spite of a greatly increased food intake is almost pathognomonic of hyperthyroidism. The links between changes in metabolic rate and changes in hunger and food intake have yet to be determined.

Certain obese patients, who, it must be emphasised, form but a very small proportion of the whole population of obese subjects, have been found under carefully controlled conditions to have a lower than normal metabolic rate. Even restricting their intake to 4.4 MJ (1000 cals) per day is insufficient to produce weight loss, as their energy expenditure is even lower. It would appear that in those patients the regulating links between food intake and energy expenditure have been overcome by the social determinants of what constitutes a normal food intake, which in western society is well above 4.4 MJ per day.

The pharmacology of drugs affecting appetite

Drugs affecting appetite and food intake fall sharply into two groups:

1 Those which reduce hunger – appetite suppressants or *anorectics*
2 Those which increase hunger

Appetite-suppressant drugs

These are of three main types:

1 Drugs acting primarily on the central nervous system
2 Drugs influencing carbohydrate metabolism
3 Bulk agents acting directly on the gastrointestinal tract

1 *Centrally acting compounds*

DRUGS ACTING ON CATECHOLAMINES

(a) *Amphetamine* This was the first anorectic compound to be introduced into clinical practice, and has been the most widely studied from the pharmacological point of view. Its anorectic action was noted as a chance finding in patients who had been prescribed the drug for narcolepsy. In fact the use of amphetamine as a stimulant in narcolepsy only came after a similar chance

241

observation that when prescribed as a nasal decongestant (its original indication) it had a stimulant activity.

In man amphetamine has a well-documented anorectic effect and has been widely used in the treatment of obesity. Unfortunately its stimulant activity has led to misuse and the drug has largely been withdrawn for use in obesity. Nevertheless its pharmacology continues to be studied enthusiastically as it has a number of psychopharmacological properties of great interest. These include the stimulant activity already referred to, a euphoriant action, an anorectic effect and a peripheral sympathomimetic action. In addition large doses can produce a paranoid psychosis closely resembling paranoid schizophrenia (see chapter 6). Therefore examination of its mode of action within the central nervous system could well increase our understanding of the central mechanisms underlying hunger, mood, arousal and psychosis; those relating to mood and psychosis being particularly relevant to psychiatry.

It is currently believed that the central effects of amphetamine depend on its actions on the catecholamine pathways within the brain (see Figure 1, p. 12).

Amphetamine, particularly the dextrorotatory (+) isomer, releases preformed NA and DA from the nerve terminals, and to a lesser extent blocks their active reuptake. There is some evidence in both man and experimental animals that the euphoriant and stimulant activity of amphetamine is mediated by DA pathways, as the effects are blocked by specific DA receptor blocking drugs such as pimozide (see chapter 6). Its anorectic action on the other hand is thought to be mediated by the ventral NA pathway, as destruction of this pathway in rats attenuates the anorectic effect of amphetamine, and in man NA receptor blockade by thymoxamine also reduces amphetamine anorexia.

Amphetamine psychosis is more fully discussed in chapters 6 and 10, suffice it to say here that this might well be mediated via a dopamine pathway involving the limbic cortex.

The sympathomimetic activity of amphetamine gives rise to cardiovascular symptoms (palpitations), dry mouth and dilatation of the pupil.

The subject of amphetamine abuse is covered in chapter 10.

(b) *Phenmetrazine, phentermine and diethylpropion* All three of these compounds have some central stimulant activity as well as an anorectic one. This is particularly pronounced in the case of phenmetrazine which has been used, like amphetamine, as a drug of abuse. The other two drugs, phentermine and diethylpropion while showing stimulant activity under laboratory conditions, for example they both increase critical flicker frequency (see chapter 4), have not been so prone to abuse. Nevertheless in many countries one or more of these drugs is subjected to the same legislative restrictions as amphetamine.

The central pharmacology of this group of drugs is similar to amphetamine, they appear to act on the catecholamine systems in the brain. It may be, however, that phentermine and diethyl-propion have a greater relative effect on NA as compared to DA pathways, and thus have less stimulant and euphoriant activity than amphetamine for an equipotent anorectic dose. This sugges-tion would explain some of the differences between them. It should be pointed out that both drugs can cause an amphetamine-like psychosis although the number of reported cases of psychosis is extremely small compared to the number of prescriptions issued.

(c) *Mazindol* It acts on both NA and DA pathways by preventing reuptake; whether or not it has a similar action on 5–HT pathways is uncertain.

DRUGS AFFECTING 5-HYDROXYTRYPTAMINE

(a) *Fenfluramine* Although chemically similar to amphetamine, and although showing an anorectic activity, fenfluramine has sedative rather than stimulant properties and has been associated with a depression of mood rather than an elevation. It is thought to act primarily on the 5–HT pathways rather than NA or DA. In animals the anorectic action of fenfluramine is impaired by drugs such as methysergide and cyproheptadine which block 5-HT receptors and by drugs which destroy 5–HT containing neurones, such as 5, 6-dihydroxytryptamine.

Not only does the neurochemical basis of fenfluramine's anorectic action differ from that of amphetamine, but its effects on the eating behaviour of rats also differs. Whereas amphetamine delays the onset of eating, fenfluramine reduces the size of the meal without affecting its onset. In man, however, experimental studies have yielded rather different results; no difference in feeding

243

pattern was observed after equivalent doses of dextroamphetamine and fenfluramine.

Fenfluramine has a peripheral action as well as a central one; it increases the uptake of glucose into muscle cells. This peripheral effect may play a part in its efficacy in treating obesity (see below).

It has recently become clear that the total anorectic activity of the racemic mixture of dl-fenfluramine resides in the d-isomer.

(b) *5–HT reuptake inhibitors* Certain new antidepressant drugs, such as fluoxetine and fluvoxamine, which act by selectively inhibiting the reuptake of 5–HT into the pre-synaptic neurone, have been noted to cause weight loss in depressed patients. This is believed to be the consequence of an increased availability of 5–HT in the synapse; 5–HT reuptake blocking drugs have the opposite effect, they increase appetite (see below).

2   *Drugs affecting carbohydrate metabolism*

(a) *Glucagon* This is a hormone produced by the α cells of the pancreas which elevates blood-sugar levels and increases the a/v glucose gradient.

While glucagon does lead to a reduction in both subjective hunger and food intake in healthy subjects as would be predicted by the glucostatic theory, the maximum effect is not observed until some two hours following intramuscular injection, occurring later than the blood-sugar effect. It may be that glucagon influences some other factor, such as gastric motility, but again the maximum reduction in motility occurs rather earlier than the maximum hunger reduction.

(b) *Biguanides* Two compounds in this group, metformin (Glucophage) and phenformin (Dibotin), which have a hypo-glycaemic action, are widely used in the treatment of diabetes mellitus, particularly the maturity-onset type commonly associated with obesity. It was noticed that obese diabetic patients appeared to lose weight much more easily while they were taking metformin or phenformin than on diet alone.

The mechanism by which these compounds affect body weight is obscure. In diabetics they increase the peripheral utilisation of glucose by improving the insulin clearance in muscle as compared to adipose tissue. Yet in non-diabetic obese subjects, where there is also a reduced peripheral glucose uptake, the biguanides do not improve peripheral glucose uptake, but probably act by reducing gluconeogenesis. It is debatable whether the biguanide compounds have a true anorectic action, as distinct from producing nausea.

3 *Opioid inhibitors* Naloxone, a relatively specific opioid receptor antagonist, when given in single doses by intramuscular injection, has been found to reduce food intake, especially intake of preferred foods, in normal subjects and in obese patients. Unfortunately longer-term treatment with naltrexone given orally had no significant effect on body weight.

4 *Bulk agents* As methylcellulose was observed to swell in the presence of water it was hoped that if it were swallowed it would similarly swell inside the stomach and thereby produce a feeling of satiety. No direct evidence of any such effect has been produced. In a series of carefully controlled observations, doses of methyl-cellulose of up to 3 g (9 tablets) led to no detectable reduction of either measured food intake or subjective hunger ratings. Equally, controlled clinical trials of these substances in obese subjects have failed to reveal any significant weight reduction attributable to them.

Appetite-stimulating drugs

1 *Insulin* Both exogenous insulin administration and endogenous hypersecretion, as occurs in spontaneous hypoglycaemia, are accompanied by a marked increase in subjective hunger. From experimental studies it is clear that this hunger does not appear until the blood sugar has reached its lowest point and is beginning to rise, that is, some thirty minutes after administration. It may be of significance that the onset of hunger occurs at approximately the same time as the appearance of pronounced fasting gastric motility. However, it is likely that both the subjective awareness of hunger and the occurrence of gastric motility are themselves secondary to hypothalamic activity.

2 *Phenothiazines* Chlorpromazine (Largactil) and its derivatives, which are widely used in the treatment of schizophrenia (see chapter 6), frequently lead to considerable weight gain; in some

series virtually all patients on continuous phenothiazine medication were noted to have gained weight, with some becoming distinctly obese. Those who develop marked adiposity report that the medication seems to make them feel voraciously hungry.

As careful studies have failed to reveal any metabolic cause for the increase in weight observed, it is likely that these compounds directly affect the hunger-regulating mechanism in the hypothalamus. Recent experimental evidence supports this view; direct injection of chlorpromazine into the lateral hypothalamus promoted increased food intake in animals.

5–HT receptor blocking drugs

(a) *Cyproheptadine (Periactin)* This compound, which has antihistaminic properties and which also antagonises the activity of 5-hydroxytryptamine, was introduced clinically as an antihistamine. Patients receiving it were noted to gain weight and laboratory animals were shown to consume more calories when cyproheptadine was given. In addition, significant weight gain was observed in both children and adults following cyproheptadine administration, as compared to that occurring after placebo. The assumption was made that the observed increase in weight reflected an underlying rise in hunger, and a consequent increase in food intake. Evidence has been obtained which substantiates this view; a group of young adults were shown to feel significantly more hungry when taking cyproheptadine than when taking placebo. This effect could be related to the compound's anti-5–HT activity, particularly as 5–HT occurs in the hypothalamus in high concentration.

(b) *Metergoline* This rather more selective 5–HT receptor blocker has been found to increase the intake of sweet foods preferentially; it had less effect on non-sweet food. The increased intake of sweet food was reversed by d-fenfluramine, a drug which increases the available 5–HT in the synapse (see above). These findings implicate 5–HT pathways in food selection as well as overall consumption.

Drug treatment of appetite disorders

The clinical conditions in which disturbances of body weight and appetite are of primary importance are obesity, psychogenic malnutrition (anorexia nervosa) and bulimia. In obesity there is an excess of adipose tissue, arising from more calories being consumed than are expended, while psychogenic malnutrition develops if more calories are expended than are consumed. The rational treatment of each situation is to reverse the calorie imbalance which has occurred. In both situations it is the appropriate dietary regime which is of fundamental importance; the place of drugs is secondary, they should only be used as adjuncts to dietary treatment, never as a substitute for it. In bulimia there is usually little if any overall calorie imbalance. The abnormality is limited to eating behaviour with body weight generally remaining constant (see below).

Obesity

For most clinical purposes body weight will suffice as an index of the degree of adiposity present; an individual can be considered as clinically obese if he exceeds his ideal body weight by 30 per cent. When this level of overweight is reached it is time for treatment to be instituted. Treatment should be based on appropriate dietary advice, together with detailed instructions, individually tailored to meet the needs and tastes of each patient, on how best to modify his or her behaviour so as to minimise the risk of non-compliance. In most cases patients will require close supervision and support which is best provided by their family doctor seeing them initially at weekly or fortnightly intervals. Such supportive care is particularly important in those patients whose obesity is a consequence of psychological disturbance. Although such patients form a minority of the overweight subjects in the population they are usually the ones who find it the most difficult to keep to a diet. Their eating pattern is not only determined by physiological requirements; psychological needs play a great part. They find that food, particularly sweet food, helps to reduce their anxiety or depression and therefore suffer greater temptations to break their diet than the majority of obese patients who have no such underlying psychological disturbance.

Appetite suppressant drugs can in some cases provide a useful

247

addition to combined dietary, behavioural and supportive treatment, but should not be used as the sole treatment.

Although amphetamine was the first centrally acting anorectic drug to be introduced, its central stimulant and euphoriant properties led to it becoming a drug of abuse (see chapter 10). Because of this most authorities now recommend that amphetamine (Benzedrine) and its dextro-isomer (Dexedrine) should not be used in the treatment of obesity; particularly as more satisfactory alternatives are now available. The same strictures apply to phenmetrazine (Preludin).

1 *Diethylpropion (Tenuate, Apisate)* While diethylpropion has an anorectic effect equal to that of amphetamine, clinically it does not appear to produce the same degree of central stimulation as amphetamine or phenmetrazine. Equally the risk of drug dependence seems to be less. Nevertheless, there is good experimental evidence to suggest that it can have a stimulant effect on the CNS as measured by CFF, and caution should therefore be applied when prescribing it.

Several controlled studies have revealed its efficacy in the treatment of obesity with daily weight losses of 20–80 g being directly attributable to the anorectic effect produced. It has been shown to be most effective when taken in doses of 50 mg one and one-half to two hours before meals. Equally effective clinically is the long-acting preparation (Tenuate dospan) which contains 75 mg diethylpropion in a slow release form.

Intermittent treatment, with alternating months on diethylpropion and placebo, has proved almost as effective as continuous treatment. As such a regime reduces the likelihood of drug dependence, it is to be preferred to continuous medication.

2 *Phentermine* Phentermine when prescribed intermittently (30 mg daily) over a period of 36 weeks was found to be as effective, in terms of weight loss, as continuous administration, and more effective than placebo.

3 *Mazindol (Teronac, Sanorex)* This drug possesses a definite, relatively long-lasting anorectic action which has proved useful in the treatment of obesity. The recommended dose is 2 mg daily given orally in the morning. Whether or not it has any advantages over diethylpropion or phentermine is uncertain, as pronounced

sympathomimetic effects and some central stimulant activity have been reported.

4 *Fenfluramine (Ponderax)* Clinically, fenfluramine (in doses of 40–120 mg daily) is an effective adjunct to weight reduction regimes, being associated with weight losses similar to those of the other compounds previously discussed. Its main distinction from those compounds is its complete lack of any stimulant properties; if anything, it has a mild sedative action which is particularly useful in the treatment of those obese patients who also show signs of anxiety. Unfortunately it too has drawbacks, being prone to produce gastrointestinal side effects, particularly diarrhoea, and acute confusional states following fenfluramine administration have been observed, particularly among patients who were receiving monoamine oxidase inhibitors at the same time. It is important to note that sudden withdrawal of fenfluramine can lead to overt depression. Reduction of dosage should therefore be undertaken gradually, and intermittent treatment with fenfluramine is not advised. In order to obtain the optimum effect it may be necessary to increase the dose in a step-wise manner to the limit of tolerance. This is because it has been shown that persistent suppression of food intake, and thus continued weight loss, occurs most consistently when the plasma level of fenfluramine exceeds 200 ng/ml.

Results of clinical trials suggest that d-fenfluramine (Isomeride) (see above) is as effective as dl-fenfluramine and is twice as potent in helping obese patients lose weight, with less tendency to cause side effects.

5 *Biguanide compounds – Metformin (Glucophage)* While this compound certainly assists obese diabetics in losing weight, its place in the treatment of uncomplicated obesity is still uncertain. At present its use should be restricted to those obese patients who are also suffering from diabetes mellitus, or who are thought to be pre-diabetic; for those patients a biguanide would appear to be the treatment of choice. The recommended dose of metformin is 0.5–1.0 g, three times daily.

6 *Bulk agents – Methylcellulose (Cellevac, Cellucon)* As there is no reliable clinical or experimental evidence to substantiate the claim

that methylcellulose reduces hunger or food intake, preparations containing methylcellulose have little place in the treatment of obesity.

7   *General recommendations*   It cannot be stressed too strongly or too often that successful weight reduction can only result from reducing intake of calories to a level below that expended. All the preparations discussed above can therefore only be considered as possible adjuncts to a sensible dietary programme and never as complete treatments in themselves. Furthermore, they should only be administered to those patients whose obesity is of clinical significance either in terms of the degree of adiposity or in the presence of serious associated disorders such as hypertension or diabetes.

With these provisos fenfluramine (particularly d-fenfluramine) appears the best suitable centrally acting appetite suppressant for general clinical use in the management of obesity. Obese diabetics may benefit more from one of the biguanide compounds.

In some quarters the use of anorectic drugs in the management of obesity is criticised on a number of counts. These include: the likelihood of pharmacological tolerance developing to the appetite-suppressant drug with consequent loss of efficacy; the high risk of inducing drug dependence; the potential these drugs have for abuse. Despite such theoretical objections, in practice there is little evidence that pharmacological tolerance actually occurs, the risk of dependence is slight and obese patients almost never resort to frank abuse of appetite-suppressant drugs. In fact, surveys of obese patients reveal that a majority of patients find the drugs useful in helping them keep to a reduced diet and thus lose weight, at least in the short term. For how long they should be prescribed is still a matter of debate; it may be that some patients would benefit from more prolonged treatment.

Anorexia nervosa (psychogenic malnutrition)

Anorexia nervosa is a condition in which severe malnutrition occurs as a result of a deliberate attempt by the patient to lose weight, usually because of pathological fear of being fat. This characteristically takes the form of drastic reduction in calorie intake, although self-induced vomiting or frequent purgation may also be practised.

Anorexia nervosa most often begins during adolescence or in early adult life, affecting females far more frequently than males. In girls, amenorrhoea supervenes sooner or later. Despite the name of the condition, appetite is preserved in many cases. The emaciation produced, although alarming, is completely reversible by dietary measures.

The place of drugs in this condition, if any, is to assist the patient to keep to the diet and thereby gain weight. Apart from general sedation which may be required in the case of a particularly uncooperative patient, certain drugs are considered by some to have a particular value in helping patients to gain weight; these include ꞌhlorpromazine, cyproheptadine and certain antidepressants.

1 *Chlorpromazine (Largactil)* Chlorpromazine and to a lesser degree other phenothiazine derivatives frequently increase appetite and produce weight gain in psychiatric patients requiring to take them over long periods. In addition they have a marked sedative effect. It is just this combination of hunger stimulation and sedation which is particularly suitable for anorexia nervosa. In many patients, however, no such medication is required as they readily settle in hospital and regain their appetite spontaneously, if they ever lose it. For those who do not respond to such relatively simple measures, chlorpromazine can be prescribed in doses from 100 mg three times daily, increasing to the level of tolerance. Care must be taken to avoid over-sedation, and the occurrence of parkinsonian symptoms will require appropriate antiparkinsonian medication, together with a reduction in dosage of chlorpromazine.

A complication observed in some 10 per cent of the patients receiving chlorpromazine for anorexia nervosa is grand mal epilepsy.

2 *Cyproheptadine* While earlier controlled trials of cyproheptadine revealed it to be of only doubtful benefit in the management of anorexia nervosa, a more recent comprehensive study has shown it to be of value as an adjunct to dietary treatment in patients whose illness is not complicated by bulimic episodes. Should bulima be present cyproheptadine is of little value.

3 *Antidepressants* Amitriptyline, in particular, possibly because of its appetite-promoting properties (see chapter 7), has been tried as

CLINICAL APPLICATIONS

a specific treatment for anorexia nervosa. While it may increase the rate of weight gain when given in association with a supervised dietary and behavioural programme, anticholinergic side effects make it less acceptable to most patients than cyproheptadine.

Bulimia nervosa

This is defined as recurrent episodes of binge eating (i.e. rapid consumption of a large amount of food in a relatively short period of time) followed by self-induced vomiting and/or purgation. It typically occurs in women who are overwhelmingly preoccupied with their body weight and shape. When it forms part of the syndrome of anorexia nervosa it carries a poor prognosis. However, the majority of patients who exhibit this behaviour are within the normal limits of body weight and, unlike women with anorexia nervosa, have a normal menstrual cycle and active sex life.

While the most effective line of treatment is based on a cognitive behavioural approach, drugs have been used successfully as adjuncts to this approach. The centrally acting appetite suppressant fenfluramine has been shown to reduce bingeing behaviour, at least in the short term. Similarly, the antidepressant drug, desipramine, has also been reported as being of benefit.

Suggestions for further reading

Regulation of food intake and pharmacology of appetite

BLUNDELL, J. E., 'Psychopharmacology of centrally acting anorectic agents', in *Psychopharmacology and Food*, ed. M. Sander and T. Silverstone, Oxford University Press, Oxford, 1985, pp. 71–109.

ROLLS, E. T., 'The neurophysiology of feeding', in *Psychopharmacology and Food*, ed. M. Sander and T. Silverstone, Oxford University Press, Oxford, 1985, pp. 1–16.

SILVERSTONE, T., 'The clinical pharmacology of appetite – its relevance to psychiatry', *Psychological Medicine*, vol. 13, 1983, pp. 251–3.

SILVERSTONE, T., and GOODALL, E., 'Serotonergic mechanisms in human feeding', *Appetite*, vol. 7, 1986, Supplement, pp. 85–97.

SMITH, G. P., 'The physiology of the meal', in *Drugs and Appetite*, ed. T. Silverstone, Academic Press, London, 1982, pp. 1–22.

TRENCHARD, E., and SILVERSTONE, T., 'Naloxone reduces the food intake of normal human volunteers', *Appetite*, vol. 4, 1983, pp. 43–50.

Drugs in the treatment of disorders of appetite and body weight

HALMI, K. A., ECKERT, E., LA DU, J. J., and COHEN, J., 'Anorexia nervosa: treatment efficacy of cyproheptadine and amitriptyline', *Archives of General Psychiatry*, vol. 43, 1986, pp. 177–81.

HUGHES, P. L., WELLS, L. A., CUNNINGHAM, C. J., and ILSTRUP, D. M., 'Treating bulimia with desipramine', *Archives of General Psychiatry*, vol. 43, 1986, pp. 182–6.

MUNRO, J. F., and FORD, M. J., 'Drug treatment of obesity', in *Drugs and Appetite*, ed. T. Silverstone, Academic Press, London, 1982, pp. 125–57.

RUSSELL, G. F. M., 'Do drugs have a place in the management of anorexia nervosa and bulimia nervosa?', in *Psychopharmacology and Food*, ed. M. Sander and T. Silverstone, Oxford University Press, Oxford, 1985, pp. 146–61.

Centrally acting drugs in the elderly

13

Elderly patients are more sensitive than are the young to the action of drugs in general, and centrally acting drugs in particular, and are more likely to develop adverse reactions to them. This must be attributable either to altered handling of the drug by the body, or to an altered effect on the body by the drug. Our knowledge of these alterations is incomplete, but this should not deter the physician from taking simple measures to improve the safety of drug treatment in his elderly patients. The most obvious of these measures are (a) avoidance of unnecessary medication; (b) improvement of patient compliance; (c) avoidance of multiple drug regimens.

Avoidance of unnecessary medication

With advancing years patients tend to be prescribed an ever increasing number of different drugs. This can only partly be explained on the basis of a true increase in pathology; in many cases drugs are prescribed for non-pathological changes which occur naturally as part of the aging process, such as the reduction in sleep requirement. It is very rarely justified to prescribe a hypnotic drug to an elderly patient other than during a major emotional crisis, and then only for a short period. There are three reasons for avoiding hypnotics in the elderly. First, old people are more susceptible to the central depressant effects of sedative drugs and, as a consequence, may show signs of a mild confusional state if they awake during the night. This is a common occurrence in hospital, brought about by the combination of strange surroundings and the overenthusiastic prescription of hypnotic drugs. It is not good practice to prescribe hypnotics routinely for all patients coming into hospital. Second, marked day-time drowsiness is a frequent problem as the rate of metabolism of these drugs is reduced in the elderly (see below). Third, there is the risk of physical dependence developing (see chapter 8). Similarly, anti-anxiety drugs are rarely required in later life. Anxiety presenting for the first time in this age group is most often a reflection of an underlying depressive illness which requires appropriate treatment in its own right (see section below on management of depression in the elderly). Furthermore, as most antianxiety drugs are benzo-diazepine compounds, the potential problems of oversedation, confusion and dependence arise here as with hypnotic drugs. Despite this over 20 per cent of women aged 65 or more in some countries report having taken antianxiety or sedative drugs during the previous year (see chapter 5), a sizeable number taking such drugs regularly.

The question whether drug treatment in early dementia is likely to be of benefit is discussed fully in chapter 9; suffice it to say here that the evidence for any such benefit is tenuous at best.

Improvement of compliance

Patients of all ages may take prescribed drugs erratically or not at all, but the elderly are particularly likely to show poor compliance with their treatment. Possible reasons for this include impaired memory, poor eyesight, polypharmacy and supervision by more than one doctor in hospital and general practice.

Compliance may be improved in several ways. Unnecessary drugs (see above) should be stopped, and the need for the remaining medication reviewed regularly. The drug regimen should be as simple as possible, with doses being given only once or twice daily. A relative, or community nurse may be asked to supervise drug administration if the patient has consented to this. Confusion among doctors supervising the patient could be reduced by the patient carrying a single medication card on which an up-to-date record of treatment could be made whenever a change is made. Alternatively, the patient should be instructed to take all his medication for inspection whenever he visits his hospital doctor or general practitioner.

Avoidance of multiple drug regimens

Many centrally acting drugs produce effects which summate when they are given together. For example, sedation may be increased if benzodiazepines are given to patients already receiving neuroleptic drugs or some antidepressants such amitriptyline or mianserin. The anticholinergic properties of antidepressants, neuroleptics and antiparkinsonian drugs may also combine to produce a syndrome characterised by delerium and clinical signs of cholinergic blockade. Furthermore, drugs given for a psychiatric indication may interact with treatment for other indications (see pages 48, 51). Constant vigilance is needed to keep the risks of treatment at an acceptable level.

Aging and the pharmacology of psychotropic drugs

Consideration of the effects of aging on the action of drugs must include two different aspects which are implicit in the definition of clinical pharmacology as the study of what drugs do to the human body, and what the body does to drugs, both in health and disease. The first part of the definition refers to the *pharmacodynamic* aspect and, in the context of this chapter, is concerned with the effects of aging on the body's response to a drug's pharmacological action. The second is concerned with the *pharmacokinetic* aspect, the influence of age on absorption, disposition and excretion of a drug (see pages 41–54). It is sometimes difficult to isolate the kinetic from the dynamic influences in a particular observed change in a drug's action associated with the aging process; nevertheless, it is convenient to approach this subject by dealing with these two aspects in turn.

There are important problems associated with studying the influence of aging on drug action in man.

1 There is the ethical problem of repeated sampling of elderly patients when the studies have no direct therapeutic value to them.
2 It may be difficult to dissociate the effects of age from those of other age-related factors such as smoking habits and intake of alcohol and caffeine which themselves may influence drug metabolism.

Influence of aging on the pharmacokinetics of psychotropic drugs

The influence of pharmacokinetics on drug action in general has been discussed elsewhere (pages 000-00). The influence of age on the various factors involved will be considered here.

1 *Absorption* There is no real evidence that drug absorption changes with increasing age, even though changes in transit time, gut pH and blood supply may occur. Recent claims that the absorptive area of the small bowel mucosa is reduced in elderly patients are not reflected in reduced absorption of psychotropic drugs, probably because of their relatively high lipid solubility and consequent easy passive diffusion across the mucosa.

2 *Distribution* Increasing age is associated with changes in body composition as well as with a general tendency to a decrease in body weight. The former may well influence the volume of distribution and compartmental distribution of some drugs, but there is little information available to document this. A decrease in body weight with age will result in higher plasma and tissue levels for a given dose of drug, but this factor is probably of lesser importance with psychotropic drugs than changes in metabolism and clearance with increasing age.

3 *Metabolism* Important changes in hepatic metabolism occur with increasing age. In an early study on this subject, amylobarbitone metabolism was compared in groups of young and elderly subjects. The excretion of 3-hydroxyamylobarbitone, an important hepatic metabolite of amylobarbitone, was significantly lower in the elderly group, but they had significantly higher plasma levels of the parent drug. These observations have been confirmed with other drugs which undergo extreme hepatic metabolism, many of them psychotropic drugs. Examples of prolonged elimination half-lives and reduced clearances for such drugs are given in Table 13.

It is difficult to be certain to what extent the reduction in hepatic metabolism of these drugs is due to a progressive age-related impairment of hepatocyte function, or to a reduction in hepatic drug uptake secondary to a reduction in liver blood flow with increasing age. Both processes probably contribute in many cases.

4 *Renal excretion* Glomerular filtration rate falls with age, even in apparently healthy subjects, and it is not surprising, therefore, that accumulation can occur of drugs which are principally excreted unchanged by the kidney. Lithium is the most important example of this among psychotropic agents, and smaller initial and maintenance doses should be used in elderly patients because of

Table 13 *Pharmacokinetic values for some hepatically metabolised psychotropic drugs in young and older subjects*

| Drug | Young (under 50 years) | | Old (over 50 years) | |
	Mean elimination half-life (hours)	Mean plasma clearance	Mean elimination half-life (hours)	Mean plasma clearance
brotizolam	5	109 ml/min	10	40 ml/min
chlordiazepoxide	10	36 ml/h/kg	18	24 ml/h/kg
clobazam	23	0.6 ml/min	48	0.4 ml/min/kg
diazepam	20	25 ml/min	90	25 ml/min
desmethyldiazepam	51	11 ml/min	151	4 ml/min
lorazepam	14	59 ml/h/kg	16	47 ml/h/kg
triazolam	3	7.5 ml/min/kg	4	3.5 ml/min/kg

their reduced renal clearance of the drug. Studies have suggested that mean weight-related daily doses should decrease by about 50 per cent between the third and eighth decades.

Influence of aging on the dynamics of psychotropic drugs

There is general agreement that older patients are more sensitive than younger to administration of centrally acting drugs, but the extent to which this is due to increased sensitivity of the brain rather than to the pharmacokinetic changes already described is uncertain. The subject is difficult to research because elderly subjects tend to perform less well in psychopharmacological tests than younger subjects even without drugs, reflecting the general deterioration in intellectual function that accompanies aging. However, there is good evidence that for a given plasma concentration of a central depressant drug such as nitrazepam, elderly subjects show more impairment of psychomotor function than do younger subjects.

If the aging brain is indeed more sensitive to action of central depressant drugs, the extent to which this is due to primary aging changes within the neurone or secondary to reduced cerebral oxygenation due to a reduction in central blood flow is uncertain.

Drug prescribing in the elderly

Clinical implications

The three psychiatric conditions occurring in later life which can present particular problems in management are depressive illness, paranoid psychosis (late paraphrenia) and confusional states.

1 *Depressive illness in the elderly* Depression in the elderly is often compounded with physical ill-health, impaired cognitive processes and adverse social circumstances. Hence, even with effective treatment the illness is likely to run a chronic course, with only a third of patients recovering by the end of a year. Furthermore, diagnosis can be difficult with the impairment of cognition accompanying depressive illness in the elderly ('pseudo-dementia') leading to a misclassification of the patient as being demented. In addition, as happens quite often, depression and dementia may coexist as independent syndromes, making the assessment of the contribution of each to the presenting psychopathology difficult. Finally, many of the treatments for the physical illnesses to which the elderly are prone can cause depressive symptoms; drugs such as alpha-methyldopa, clonidine and reserpine are particularly likely to do this. Here, adjusting or substituting the medication is the appropriate first step in the treatment of the affective disturbance.

Antidepressant drugs (see chapter 7) are generally as effective in the treatment of depressive illness in the elderly as in younger patients although complete resolution of symptoms may be less frequently achieved. The choice of antidepressant for use in elderly depressives depends largely on the side effects of the different preparations. As older patients are prone to ischaemic heart disease and, in the case of males, prostatic hypertrophy, it is necessary to choose an antidepressant drug with low cardiotoxic potential and little anticholinergic activity. Furthermore, anticholinergic drugs have been implicated as a cause of deterioration of cognitive function. While mianserin and trazadone fulfil these requirements and are thus widely used in the elderly, mianserin's pronounced sedative effect makes it unacceptable to many. Possible alternatives are dothiepin and lofepramine (see chapter 8).

Elderly patients who present with a pronounced hypochondriacal

259

element to their depressive illness often benefit from treatment with a monoamine oxidase inhibitor (MAOI) such as phenelzine. The dose should be increased cautiously and the necessary dietary restrictions strictly adhered to (see chapter 8). With these provisos there is no particular contraindication to MAOI in the elderly. In fact, many previously resistant depressions respond to MAOI. If this fails, ECT may be indicated. Where psychomotor retardation is pronounced ECT is often the treatment of choice.

The frequency of recurrent depression in the elderly can be reduced by prophylactic long-term lithium. Close and regular attention must be paid to renal function (see above) and to thyroid status.

2 *Late paraphrenia* Late paraphrenia is a form of schizophrenia characterised by a well-systematised paranoid delusional state having its onset in late life. Women are more frequently affected than men, particularly single women living alone whose hearing is impaired.

The paranoid symptoms usually respond well initially to antipsychotic drugs (see chapter 6). But relapse is frequent, usually as a consequence of the patient failing to continue taking the prescribed medication. No single antipsychotic has proved more effective than any other; choice depends on side effects. While thioridazine, perhaps the most commonly prescribed antipsychotic for elderly patients, is less likely to cause extrapyramidal symptoms because of its additional anticholinergic properties, it is particularly prone to precipitate postural hypotension due to its noradrenergic blocking action. Trifluperazine has also been widely used. Pimozide may possess a potential advantage in that it requires less frequent administration, thus failure to comply may prove less of a problem, provided a family member or a community psychiatric nurse can ensure that at least one dose per week is taken. Depot injections are another useful alternative for the otherwise non-compliant patient who is willing to accept them.

Tardive dyskinesia (see chapter 6) is particularly prevalent in the elderly, so dosage must be kept to the minimum to avoid it.

3 *Confusional states* Elderly patients frequently show signs of an acute confusional state during the course of an acute physical illness, following a surgical operation, or as a result of heavy-handed administration of sedatives. Recovery from the underlying

illness usually results in complete resolution of the psychiatric disorder and initial treatment must be directed towards the underlying cause. Occasionally, where behaviour is so disturbed as to make nursing difficult, it may be necessary to use a centrally acting drug such as chlorpromazine, but this must be used with caution and circumspection (see chapter 9). Where the syndrome is thought to be drug-induced, nursing care in an appropriate environment until the effects of the drug wear off is usually all that is required.

Confusion is an integral part of the clinical syndrome of dementia. Unfortunately there are as yet no definitive treatments for the various types of dementia. The management of any associated disturbance of behaviour is fully described in chapter 9; essentially it is based on the judicious administration of thioridazine or haloperidol.

Suggestions for further reading

ABOU-SALEH, M. T., and COPPEN, A., 'The prognosis of depression in old age – the case for lithium therapy', *British Journal of Psychiatry*, vol. 143, 1983, pp. 527–8.

CASTLEDEN, D. M., GEORGE, C. F., MARCER, D., and HALLETT, C., 'Increased sensitivity to nitrazepam in old age', *British Medical Journal*, vol. 1, 1977, pp. 10–12.

EISDORFER, C., and FAN, W. E., *Psychopharmacology of Aging*, MTP, Lancaster, 1980.

GERNER, R., 'Present status of drug therapy of depression in later life', *Journal of Affective Disorders*, Supplement 1, 1985, pp. 523–31.

GRAHAME, P. S., 'Late paraphrenia', *British Journal of Hospital Medicine*, vol. X, 1982, pp. 522–8.

HEWICK, D. S., NEWBUG, P., HOPWOOD, S., NAYLOR, G., and MOODY, J., 'Age as a factor affecting lithium therapy', *British Journal of Clinical Pharmacology*, vol. 4, 1977, pp. 201–5.

IRVINE, R. E., GROVE, J., TOSELAND, P. A., and TROUNCE, J. A., 'The effect of age on the hydroxylation of amylobarbitone sodium in man', *British Journal of Clinical Pharmacology*, vol. 1, 1974, pp. 41–3.

JOCHENSEN, R., NANDI, K. L., CORLESS, D., WESSELMAN, J. G. J., and BREIMAR, D. D., 'Pharmacokinetics of brotizolam in the elderly', *British Journal of Clinical Pharmacology*, vol. 16, 1983, pp. 2995–3075.

O'MALLEY, K., JUDGE, T. D., and CROOKS, J., 'Geriatric clinical pharmacology and therapeutics', in *Drug Treatment*, 2nd edn, ed. G. S. Avery, Churchill Livingstone, Edinburgh, 1980, pp. 158–81.

Child psychiatry

14

In general, drug treatment has but a limited place in child psychiatry. The majority of cases presenting to the child psychiatrist require social and psychotherapeutic support rather than pharmacological intervention. Nevertheless, there are certain syndromes which do benefit from psychotropic drugs. In general such drugs act through the control of a symptom rather than in producing any basic modification of the underlying disorder. Although there is some disagreement among child psychiatrists concerning the efficacy of drug treatment in the disorders which they treat, drugs have been used successfully in the following conditions: attention deficit disorder; behaviour disturbance in brain-damaged and epileptic children; school refusal; nocturnal enuresis; some cases of stammering; certain patients with motor tics. Those rare cases of true schizophrenia which occur during the later stages of childhood respond to neuroleptic drugs in a similar fashion to adults (see chapter 6). However, particular caution is required when prescribing antipsychotic drugs for younger patients. They are more likely than adults to experience an acute dystonic reaction and are more susceptible to drug-induced convulsions.

Attention deficit disorder (hyperkinetic syndrome)

The hyperkinetic syndrome (which is thought by some to be a reflection of underlying brain damage) is characterised by extreme restlessness and distractability, usually coming on between the ages of two and five. There may or may not be frank neurological signs. It is relatively uncommon in its severe form, although minor degrees of restlessness with short attention space, particularly in the classroom, are observed much more frequently, especially in boys. Epilepsy, which complicates the picture in a minority of cases, should be controlled with a suitable anticonvulsant.

Dexamphetamine (Dexedrine), although a stimulant drug, has a beneficial effect on hyperkinetic activity in children; an appropriate dose is 5–10 mg daily; this may be increased to a maximum of 40 mg. This is not, as is sometimes believed, a 'paradoxical' effect; what appears to be happening is that dexamphetamine improves the attention span, and consequently reduces the child's tendency to distractability. Methylphenidate (Ritalin) 10–60 mg daily is an equally effective alternative. Magnesium pemoline (Pemoline), another stimulant compound, has a long half-life which tends to give a more stable pharmacological action. While numerous controlled trials have attested to the beneficial effects of stimulant drugs on classroom behaviour in the short term, follow-up studies have failed to reveal any long-term advantages, in terms of emotional adjustment, delinquent behaviour, or academic performance, among hyperkinetic children treated with methylphenidate as compared to children not so treated. Furthermore, these drugs do have some serious potential disadvantages. First, the side effects of insomnia, tachycardia and anorexia may prove troublesome, although the insomnia can be reduced by giving the drug early in the day. Second, these drugs do impair growth, although the effect is slight and probably not permanent. Nevertheless, even mild stunting of growth could be a grave disadvantage in certain children.

It has been reported that the incidence of drug abuse is higher among those children with the hyperkinetic syndrome who have received amphetamine in the past. Thus administration of these drugs should be strictly limited to those children with unequivocal symptoms and signs of the condition. Even among these there is a very good chance that considerable improvement will occur by adolescence. It is therefore recommended that when stimulant drugs are prescribed, they should be stopped from time to time to see if they are still required.

Behaviour disturbance in brain-damaged children

It is now generally recognised that psychiatric disorder is common among children showing evidence of brain damage, the most frequent abnormality being antisocial behaviour. Other syndromes thought to be a reflection of underlying cerebral pathology include the hyperkinetic syndrome, aggressive outbursts and autistic behaviour. Many brain-damaged children also suffer from epilepsy

263

and, where this occurs, adequate control of epileptic attacks will often improve the situation considerably. Control may be achieved by phenytoin (Epanutin) 60–200 mg daily, primidone (Mysoline) 100–500 mg daily, carbamazepine (Tegretol) 100–500 mg daily, sulthiame (Ospolot) 60–300 mg daily. In addition the latter compound has been reported to improve behaviour in disturbed mentally handicapped patients who are not epileptic. As pheno-barbitone tends to exacerbate behaviour disorders it should be avoided where possible in the management of epileptic children who manifest disturbed behaviour.

In addition to epilepsy there may be other associated neuro-logical abnormalities which further complicate the life of the brain-damaged child. Thus the management of behaviour disturbance in children with brain damage encompasses rather more than just the prescription of an appropriate drug; a comprehensive social, psychological and physical approach is required. In fact one leading authority has gone so far as to state: 'The advice to those about to prescribe for the mentally handicapped is – when in doubt don't.' Drugs, when used for mentally handicapped patients, should be prescribed on the same basis as for children without such problems, and should in general be given for relatively brief periods only. If more prolonged treatment is required then repeated reassessments of the need for the drug should be made.

The behaviour of brain-damaged children may be punctuated by short-lived outbursts of extreme aggression and destructiveness. These episodic symptoms can be ameliorated by neuroleptic drugs of the phenothiazine type (e.g. chlorpromazine) or the butyro-phenone type (e.g. haloperidol). It is recommended that the use of such drugs should be limited as far as possible to controlling the outburst when it happens.

School refusal and panic attacks

The extreme reluctance to go to school displayed by some children is not so much a phobia of school itself, but rather a fear of leaving the security of the home. It must be distinguished from other causes of non-attendance at school, particularly truancy, which is a reflection of an antisocial attitude rather than of anxiety. Some authorities have suggested that the symptoms of school phobia can reflect underlying depression, which may be accompanied by such somatic symptoms as abdominal pain or headaches.

Although the majority of school refusers can be handled

successfully without recourse to drugs, in some cases, particularly when there have been panic attacks, an anxiolytic sedative of the benzodiazepine type (see chapter 8) can reduce anxiety sufficiently to allow the child to contemplate going back to school. Chlordiazepoxide (Librium) 5–10 mg two or three times daily and diazepam (Valium) 2–5 mg three times daily are both suitable. When used for this purpose the administration of benzodiazepines should be restricted to periods of crisis, rather than given continuously. As some of these children may be depressed, the administration of an antidepressant drug of the monoamine reuptake inhibiting type (MARI), such as amitriptyline 10 to 25 mg, given as a single bed-time dose may be of value. Obsessional symptoms, when they occur in childhood, appear to respond preferentially to clomipramine, as in adults (see chapter 8).

Nocturnal enuresis

Nocturnal enuresis, or bedwetting at night, can be considered abnormal if it persists after the age of five. It is now generally believed to be the result of delayed maturation, rather than secondary to emotional problems. In favour of this view is the observation that almost all enuretic children become completely dry at night by the time they leave school. As an approximation, some 15 per cent of children aged five frequently wet the bed at night; this figure falls to 5 per cent among 10-year-olds, and to 1 per cent by the age of 15. Rarely, nocturnal enuresis is a symptom of structural abnormality of the urinary tract, and in those cases there is usually incontinence by day as well as by night.

If physical examination and urinanalysis fail to reveal any abnormality, and the sole symptom is bedwetting, the condition is almost certainly primary nocturnal enuresis, and further investigation is rarely called for.

Drug treatment appears to help some children affected by this problem, although as yet no drug has been nearly as effective as conditioning treatment. This may take one of two forms, the first being the reinforcement of dry behaviour through the provision of a reward, normally approbation coupled with stars. The second type is required in the more severe cases; this involves the use of a bell and pad to continue the conditioning. Drugs, being so much easier to administer, are often used in the first instance in spite of the disadvantages of serious side effects and potential toxicity.

Probably by virtue of their associated anticholinergic effects together with their known potentiation of adrenergic activity (see chapter 2), tricyclic antidepressant drugs, such as imipramine (Tofranil), amitriptyline (Tryptizol, Elavil) and nortriptyline (Aventyl), in a dose of 25–50 mg at night, have been shown to be of greater effectiveness than placebo in reducing the frequency of bedwetting. Although this is of some benefit, they only achieve the complete remission which most patients (and their parents) seek in 20 per cent of cases. Unfortunately, relapse almost always occurs when drug treatment is stopped. Treatment with these drugs is most useful as a short-term measure to prevent bedwetting as on a school outing or when visiting a friend's house. If successful within three or four weeks then medication should be continued for at least another month before being cautiously reduced over the ensuing few months. Relapse during this time calls for raising the dose to the level at which a favourable response had been achieved.

If trycyclic drugs in adequate dosage fail to produce an adequate improvement within four weeks there is little point in persevering with this line of treatment, particularly as cases of tricyclic poisoning are increasing among children.

Stuttering (stammering)

Frequent interruption of the free flow of speech, severe enough to interfere with communication, which is made worse by conscious efforts to overcome it, characterises the condition of stuttering. While this may occur to some degree in up to 3 per cent of children, only 1 per cent become persistent stutterers. As far as drug treatment is concerned, haloperidol 0.75–1.5 mg three times a day (when combined with speech therapy) has been shown to be better than a placebo given under the same conditions. Behavioural techniques which train the child to speak in a strict rhythm (by using a metronome) are also of value. Combinations of drugs with such behaviour therapy have yet to be evaluated.

Tics

Tics may be defined as brief, jerky involuntary movements, which occur particularly in the muscles around the eyes and lower part of the face. They are relatively common, being present in up to 5 per cent of all children at some time; the time they are most likely to occur is between the ages of five and ten. Tics are usually exacerbated by emotional distress, and are more frequently found in boys. Drugs of the anxiolytic sedative type such as the benzodiazepines (e.g. chlordiazepoxide 5–10 mg or diazepam 2–5 mg three times daily) may help reduce the emotional component of the condition and thereby reduce the frequency of the tics. Haloperidol 0.5–1.5 mg three times daily has also been found to be of benefit, although the larger dose may lead to extrapyramidal effects.

Gilles de la Tourette syndrome, a condition characterised by multiple motor tics and involuntary vocalisations (see chapter 9) typically begins in childhood. As in adults, the dopamine receptor blocking drugs haloperidol and pimozide have been found to be effective in reducing symptoms in affected children.

Sleeplessness and food refusal

These two symptoms are frequent manifestations of behaviour disturbance in early childhood. Symptomatic treatment with chlorpromazine, taken as a single 50 to 100 mg dose at night, can frequently provide sufficient control of the condition to allow any necessary environmental and attitudinal changes to take place within the family. While it is important to give an effective sedative dose, side effects, particularly a light-sensitive rash, can occur. As before, drug treatment should be of limited duration, being viewed merely as a way of intervening in what has become a vicious circle of interaction between parent and child.

Anorexia nervosa

See chapter 12.

Suggestions for further reading

KAPLAN, C. A., and KOLVIN, I., 'Drugs in child psychiatry', in *Recent Advances in Clinical Psychiatry*, vol. 5, ed. K. Granville-Grossman, Churchill Livingstone, Edinburgh, 1985, pp. 161–78.

TAYLOR, E., 'Drug treatment' in *Child and Adolescent Psychiatry*, 2nd edn, ed. M. Rutter and L. Hersov, Blackwell, Oxford, 1985, pp. 780–93.

WERRY, J. S., *Pediatric Psychopharmacology*, Brunner Mazel, New York, 1978.

The management of overdosage of centrally acting drugs $\quad$ 15

Self-poisoning with centrally acting drugs, particularly hypnotics and antidepressants, is the commonest method of suicide in the United Kingdom. There are certain principles which apply to the treatment of such self-poisoning, irrespective of the actual substance ingested.

Maintenance of respiration

Respiratory depression occurs with many centrally acting drugs, particularly the barbiturates and other hypnotics. In addition, there may be airway obstruction due to inhalation of vomitus or to excessive mucus production. It is, therefore, necessary to ensure a clear airway by removing any dentures, pulling the tongue forward and removing saliva and vomitus from the mouth and pharynx. In the deeply unconscious patient with no cough reflex an endo-tracheal tube is necessary; in other patients a short oropharyngeal airway should be inserted. The patient should be turned into the semi-prone position and the adequacy of ventilation assessed. If there is any suspicion of inadequate ventilation, oxygen should be administered and assisted ventilation considered. Regular arterial blood gas analyses are the best way to assess ventilation. There is no place for the use of analeptic drugs in overdosage with psychotropic drugs. They have a narrow therapeutic ratio and may produce epileptiform convulsions and cardiac dysrhythmias.

Maintenance of cardiovascular function

Drugs may cause hypotension by a number of mechanisms including:

1 depression of the vasomotor centre;
2 direct depression of myocardial contractility;

3 increase in venous capacitance leading to reduced venous return to the heart and consequent fall in cardiac output;
4 prolonged vomiting or excessive sweating which can cause marked fluid depletion and fall in circulatory volume.

If hypotension does not respond to elevation of the foot of the bed a central venous pressure line should be inserted and colloid infused continuously to increase the circulatory volume. If this fails to reverse the hypotension, consideration should be given to the use of inotropic agents such as dopamine or dobutamine.

Many psychotropic drugs produce cardiac dysrhythmias and cardiac monitoring should, therefore, be employed where possible during the recovery period in all patients. This is particularly true for the monoamine reuptake inhibitor antidepressant drugs, where both their anticholinergic and catecholamine reuptake inhibiting properties may play a part in production of rhythm irregularities. Correction of hypoxia or acidosis may abolish dysrhythmias, but if not, careful consideration should be given to specific drug therapy, e.g. with lignocaine, remembering however that many anti-dysrhythmic drugs may potentiate the myocardial depressant effect of the drugs taken in overdose.

Control of neurological complications and convulsions

Convulsions may occur in overdosage with central stimulant and antidepressant compounds, and also in phenothiazine poisoning in which the epileptic seizure threshold is reduced. If infrequent and of short duration no specific therapy is required, but repeated or prolonged convulsions can be controlled by intravenous diazepam 10 mg repeated as necessary. If the patient is also vomiting, temporary intubation and mechanical ventilation may be necessary to prevent aspiration pneumonia.

Routine care of the unconscious patient should include assessment of the level of consciousness, and regular turning to avoid skin damage and nerve and muscle compression injuries. The bladder can often be emptied by firm suprapubic pressure, but catheterisation is necessary if this manoeuvre fails or when measurement of urine volume is important. Cerebral oedema may be caused by hypoxia, hypercapnia, hypoglycaemia or hypotension. It should be carefully looked for in patients who have sustained cardiorespiratory arrest, and treated initially with intravenous mannitol followed by dexamethasone intramuscularly.

Reduction of absorption

When it is known that the drug concerned has been ingested within four hours of admission to hospital, it is reasonable to attempt to prevent further absorption by emptying the patient's stomach or by administering actuated charcoal which adsorbs drug on to its surface. If the patient is conscious it may be possible to induce emesis by pharyngeal stimulation or administration of syrup of ipecacuanha. Certain drugs (e.g. salicylates, monoamine reuptake inhibitors, anticholinergic drugs, opiates) delay gastric emptying and lavage or emesis may be effective after more than four hours. In the unconscious patient, a cuffed endotracheal tube must always be inserted before lavage is instituted. Lavage is contraindicated if there is any suspicion that the patient may have taken corrosives or petroleum substances, and in patients known to have upper alimentary disease, because of the risk of perforation.

Enhancement of drug elimination

Forced diuresis increases the renal clearance of salicylates and phenobarbitone when the urine is alkaline, and amphetamines, fenfluramine and phencyclidine when the urine is acid.

Such patients should have normal cardiac and renal function since the diuresis is achieved by infusing large volumes of fluid intravenously. A careful assessment of fluid balance is therefore necessary, and unconscious patients require bladder catheterisation. If the fluid input exceeds the output at any stage by 2 litres or more, intravenous frusemide is given. The aim of alkaline diuresis is to maintain the urine pH between 7.0 and 8.0 (checked by indicator paper), but if large amounts of bicarbonate are needed to achieve this, the arterial pH and serum potassium and calcium should be carefully monitored. Forced acid diuresis is less frequently required. Ammonium chloride is given (either orally or intravenously) to keep urine pH below 5.0 and careful monitoring of aterial pH is also mandatory. Haemodialysis is useful in removing drugs which have low plasma protein binding, volume of distribution and lipid solubility. It is generally reserved for treatment of severe overdosage, particularly in those patients with secondary complications. Salicylates, phenobarbitone, ethanol, methanol and lithium are effectively removed by this method. Haemoperfusion of arterial blood through an extracorporeal column of activated charcoal or ion-exchange resin will effectively remove some drugs, even though their lipid solubility and/or plasma protein binding may be high. It is again reserved for severe poisoning, particularly when serious complications are present. Barbiturates, glutethimide, methaqualone ethchlorvynol, meprobamate and chloral hydrate may be effectively removed by this method. It is not of value in treatment of overdosage of monoamine reuptake inhibiting (tricyclic) antidepressive drugs.

Identification of the poison

This is important in determining subsequent management and for medicolegal and forensic purposes. If a reliable history is not available, clinical features and laboratory investigations may assist in identification of the drug(s) involved.

Psychiatric assessment and treatment

During the recovery phase, the patient may become agitated, distressed or even violent, and may require sedation.

If there is any reason to believe that the drug overdosage is the result of deliberate self-harm, then the management must include an evaluation of the psychiatric and social state. Such an evaluation need not be by a psychiatrist, but should be carried out by a medical practitioner, nurse, social worker or clinical psychologist specifically trained for the task. Every hospital should have a clearly laid down code of practice about the management of such patients.

Specific measures

In certain cases of poisoning with centrally acting drugs, additional specific measures may be indicated.

1 *Opiates* Naloxone is the narcotic antagonist of choice because it lacks partial agonist properties and so does not itself produce narcotic effects. It is given to reduce respiratory depression, and may precipitate an acute abstinence syndrome if physical dependence has developed on the narcotic drug.

2 *Monoamine oxidase inhibitors* Overdosage with these drugs may be associated with hyperpyrexia, for which chlorpromazine is the treatment of choice. If marked hypertension is present, this should be treated with an alpha-adrenoceptor blocking drug such as phentolamine or thymoxamine.

Reference centres

In many countries information on the management of cases of drug overdosage may be obtained at any time from the relevant poison information centres. For the United Kingdom the appropriate telephone numbers are given in the *British National Formulary*; for the United States they appear in the *Physicians Desk Reference*.

Suggestions for further reading

HENRY, J., 'Can tricyclic antidepressants be removed by haemoperfusion?' *Human Toxicology*, vol. 1, 1982, pp. 359–60.

HENRY, J., and VOLANS, G., *ABC of Poisoning*, British Medical Association, London, 1985.

MATTHEW, H., and LAWSON, A. A. H., *Treatment of Common Acute Poisonings*, 4th edn, Churchill Livingstone, Edinburgh, 1979.

OSSELTON, M. D., BLACKMORE, R. C., KING, L. A., and MOFFAT, A. C., 'Poisoning-associated deaths for England and Wales between 1973 and 1980', *Human Toxicology*, vol. 3, 1984, pp. 201–21.

POLSON, C. J., GREEN, M. A., and LEE, M. R., *Clinical Toxicology*, 3rd edn, Pitman, Bath, 1983.

PROUDFOOT, A., *Diagnosis and Management of Acute Poisoning*, Blackwell Scientific Publications, Oxford, 1982.

VALE, J. A., and MEREDITH, T. J., *Poisoning: Diagnosis and Treatment*, Update Books, London, 1981.

Subject Index

Index of Drug names

ABSTEM, *see* Calcium carbimide
AKINETON, *see* Biperiden
Alcohol, 3
Alpha-methyldopa, 30, 31, 34, 259
Alpha-methylparatyrosine, 30, 111
Alprazolam, 166, 188, 198, 199
Amitriptyline, 43, 45, 47, 50, 152,
    161, 175, 234, 251, 265, 266
Amoxapine, 177
Amphetamine, 31, 33, 34, 35, 42,
    46, 59, 73, 147, 154, 156, 215,
    219, 230, 234, 237, 241, 248;
    psychosis, 107
Amylobarbitone, 59
ANAFRANIL, *see* Clomipramine
ANQUIL, *see* Benperidol
ANTABUSE, *see* Disulfiram
ANXON, *see* Ketazolam
APISATE, *see* Diethylpropion
Apomorphine, 27, 36, 113
ARTANE, *see* Benzhexol
ATIVAN, *see* Lorazepam
Atropine, 11, 13, 25
AVENTYL, *see* Nortriptyline

Baclofen, 16, 129
Benperidol (Benzperidol), 136, 226
BENZEDRINE, *see* Amphetamine
Benzhexol, 13, 51, 125, 169
Biperiden, 125
BOLVIDON, *see* Mianserin
Bromazepam, 188, 199
Bromocriptine, 14, 37, 131, 166
Brotizolam, 233, 258
Buprenorphine, 218

BUSPAR, *see* Buspirone
Buspirone, 191, 197, 199
Butriptyline, 175

Caffeine, 16, 157, 195
Calcium Carbimide, 214
CAMCOLIT, *see* Lithium
Cannabis, 4, 215, 220
Carbamazepine, 160, 170, 174, 212,
    264
CELLEVAC, *see* Methylcellulose
Chloral Hydrate, 206, 234, 236
Chlorcyclizine, 15
Chlordiazepoxide, 59, 187, 188,
    199, 203, 211, 258, 265, 267
Chlormethiazole, 203, 206, 212
P-Chlorophenylalanine, 30, 230
Chlorpromazine, 5, 19, 35, 36, 37,
    110, 111, 113, 114, 117, 119, 131,
    132, 133, 153, 169, 202, 223, 237,
    245, 251, 261, 264
Chlorprothixene, 135
Cimetidine, 15
Clobazam, 188, 199, 258
Clomipramine, 36, 162, 175, 265
Clonazepam, 170
Clonidine, 37, 51, 149, 209, 259
Clopenthixol Deconoate, 135
CLOPIXOL CONCENTRATE,
    see Clopenthixol Deconoate
Clorazepate, 187, 189, 199
Clorgyline, 35, 154, 165
Clozapine, 116
Cocaine, 4, 35, 154, 215, 220
CONCORDIN, *see* Protriptyline